Library

Medical Association

Radiology Boards

Dave Maudgil
Consultant Radiologist
Heatherwood and Wexham Park Hospitals

Foreword by
Anthony Watkinson
Consultant Interventional Radiologist
The Royal Devon and Exeter Hospital

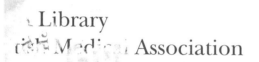

Radcliffe Publishing
Oxford • Seattle

Radcliffe Publishing Ltd
18 Marcham Road
Abingdon
Oxon OX14 1AA
United Kingdom

www.radcliffe-oxford.com
Electronic catalogue and worldwide online ordering facility.

British Library Cataloguing in Publication Data

A catalogue record for this book is available from the British Library.

ISBN 1 85775 677 0

Typeset by Advance Typesetting Ltd, Oxford
Printed and bound by TJ International Ltd, Padstow, Cornwall

Contents

Foreword

Radiologists-in-training are faced with a continually widening curriculum and ever-changing examinations. The FRCR Part 2 examination is no exception having changed radically over recent times. Not only does it span basic physics, anatomy and technique but also includes clinical and cross-sectional imaging at an advanced level.

This book is an excellent revision tool to test knowledge required to pass this exam. It is written by a newly appointed consultant who has recently passed the FRCR and who has a proven track record in teaching, having been involved in running successfully the FRCR course at the Royal Free Hospital for several years. The book provides a structured system-based approach, enabling modules to be studied and revised separately. It provides detailed explanatory text on MCQ questions and answers, enabling the candidate to test their knowledge and revise concurrently. It also includes reference texts should the candidate wish to source the information and delve deeper.

I recommend this book to all radiologists-in-training and in particular those preparing for the FRCR. I wish it every success.

Dr Anthony Watkinson FRCS FRCR
Consultant Interventional Radiologist
The Royal Devon and Exeter Hospital
Exeter, UK
January 2005

Preface

This book has been written in response to the changes in Part 2 of the FRCR examination. The examination now includes basic radiological science questions (i.e. relevant physics, anatomy and technique) as well as the original clinical imaging component and tests cross-sectional imaging, in particular, at an advanced level. The book also includes some more traditional exam favourites which crop up fairly regularly.

In terms of books for preparing for the exam, I would recommend every examinee should have Dahnert's *Radiology Review Manual* to hand for ready reference; other useful books which have been used in compiling and checking the questions are listed in the bibliography.

Several different techniques have been suggested to maximise the exam score. It is worth seeing how well you fare on your 'guesses', particularly if the exam is negatively marked. Even if your guesses are right 70% of the time, you can still score 40% versus 0% for not guessing at all.

While researching for this book it became clear that many questions would be useful for preparation for the American Board of Radiology exams.

Good luck and success in your exams and careers!

Dave Maudgil
January 2005

About the author

Dave Maudgil qualified in medicine from Guy's Hospital in 1991 and did medical SHO jobs in London. He passed his MRCP in 1994. He worked as a medical registrar at St George's Hospital, Tooting, and then as a research registrar in neurology at the National Hospital, Queen Square, and the National Society for Epilepsy in Chalfont St Peter. His project was on identifying cortical abnormalities on MRI scans of patients with epilepsy. He underwent training in radiology at the Royal Free Hospital, Hampstead, passing his FRCR in 2001. He was appointed as consultant radiologist (with an interest in interventional radiology) at Heatherwood and Wexham Park Hospitals in 2003.

Contributor

Dr C Hartigan
Specialist Registrar
Royal Free Hospital
Hampstead
London

For Uday and Megha, with love.

Section 1

Thorax

(Q1) Are the following statements regarding severe acute respiratory distress syndrome (SARS) true or false?

(a) SARS can be confidently diagnosed with a single test.
(b) It is caused by SARS-associated coronavirus.
(c) The chest radiograph (CXR) findings are easily distinguishable from those of other causes of atypical pneumonia.
(d) The right lung is more commonly affected than the left.
(e) Calcification, cavitation, pleural effusions and lymphadenopathy are common findings, particularly in the paediatric population.

(Q2) Are the following statements true or false? Bronchoalveolar carcinoma:

(a) typically occurs peripherally.
(b) may cause the computed tomography (CT) angiogram sign.
(c) occurs most commonly in a multicentric form.
(d) is negative on fluorodeoxyglucose positron emission tomography (FDG PET) in more than 50% of cases.
(e) can present with bronchorrhea.

(Q3) Cigarette smoking is associated with the following conditions. True or false?

(a) Cryptogenic fibrosing alveolitis (CFA).
(b) Non-specific interstitial pneumonitis (NSIP).
(c) Eosinophilic pneumonia.

1

(d) Langerhans cell histiocytosis (LCH).
(e) Bronchiectasis.

Q4 Are the following statements regarding ultrasound (US) of the chest true or false?

(a) The diagnosis of rib fractures is easier than on plain film.
(b) Pneumothoraces can cause a marked increase in reverberation artefact.
(c) Low resistance flow on colour Doppler helps distinguish benign from malignant tumours.
(d) A thrombosed pulmonary artery may be diagnosed via the 'vessel sign'.
(e) A linear probe is ideal.

Q5 Are the following statements regarding pulmonary thromboembolism true or false?

(a) Pulmonary thromboembolism requires gadolinium for diagnosis on magnetic resonance imaging (MRI).
(b) A focal area of pulmonary hypoperfusion may cause a false-positive diagnosis.
(c) Subsegmental emboli may be visualised with 3 mm collimation.
(d) Pulmonary hypertension predisposes to increased mortality in pulmonary angiography.
(e) In the multicentre PIOPED study, 40% of scans were classified as being of intermediate probability.

Q6 The following may occur after lung transplantation. True or false?

(a) Lung torsion at six weeks.
(b) Bronchial dehiscence.
(c) Pulmonary embolism in the acute phase.
(d) Pneumatosis intestinalis.
(e) Recurrence of sarcoidosis in the transplanted lung.

Q7 Are the following statements regarding cardiac tumours true or false?

(a) Right atrial myxomas are the commonest primary intracardiac tumours.
(b) Of rhabdomyomas, 50% occur with tuberous sclerosis.
(c) Fibromas typically calcify.
(d) Hydatid disease may cause myocardial cysts.
(e) MRI and ultrafast CT are sensitive for diagnosis.

Q8 The following are recognised causes of pericardial effusions. True or false?

(a) Post-myocardial infarction.
(b) Collagen vascular disease.
(c) Mesothelioma.
(d) Irradiation.
(e) Gout.

Q9 The following conditions are associated with ventilation–perfusion mismatch. True or false?

(a) Vasculitis.
(b) Hypoplasia of the pulmonary artery.
(c) Pleural effusion.
(d) Hilar adenopathy.
(e) BOOP (bronchiolitis obliterans with organising pneumonia).

Q10 Are the following statements regarding pericardial defects true or false?

(a) They are more common on the right side.
(b) They only occur in adults.
(c) They are associated with bronchogenic cysts.
(d) They may cause difficult visualisation of the right heart border.
(e) They require no intervention.

Q11 Are the following statements regarding myocardial perfusion imaging true or false?

(a) Thallium-205 chloride is a commonly used agent.
(b) Normally less than 5% activity of technetium-99 sestamibi remains at 10 minutes.
(c) Critical aortic stenosis is a contraindication to stress testing.
(d) The reverse distribution pattern is pathognomic of cardiac infarction.
(e) Quantitative analysis can be presented via a bull's eye display.

Q12 Are the following statements true or false? Cryptogenic organising pneumonia (COP):

(a) may be caused by extrinsic allergic alveolitis.
(b) occurs typically in the 20–40-years age group.
(c) may be preceded by a flu-like illness.
(d) occurs typically in the upper zones.
(e) improves with corticosteroids.

Q13 Chronic alveolar infiltrate may be caused by the following conditions. True or false?

(a) Lipoid pneumonia.
(b) Goodpasture's syndrome.
(c) Alveolar proteinosis.
(d) Pulmonary contusion.
(e) Alveolar cell carcinoma.

Q14 Lymphoid interstitial pneumonia is associated with the following conditions. True or false?

(a) Acquired immune deficiency syndrome (AIDS).
(b) Chronic active hepatitis.
(c) Salivary gland enlargement.
(d) Parenchymal cysts.
(e) Centrilobular nodules.

Q15 The following may cause septal lines. True or false?

(a) Pulmonary oedema.
(b) Mycoplasma pneumonia.
(c) Cryptogenic organising pneumonia.
(d) Lymphangioleiomyomatosis.
(e) Wegener's granulomatosis.

Q16 Are the following statements true or false?

(a) The transverse sinus of the pericardium is situated anterior to the ascending aortic root.
(b) The oblique sinus is in direct connection with the superior pericardial recess.
(c) In the anomalous innominate artery compression syndrome, the anterior wall of the trachea is indented by the right brachiocephalic artery.
(d) Further investigations are required in patients with a right-sided aortic arch and mirror branch imaging.
(e) The right atrium typically enlarges in a posterior direction.

Q17 Are the following statements regarding radiation pneumonitis true or false?

(a) It is most extensive at two weeks.
(b) It is always accompanied by symptoms.
(c) It may be enhanced by bleomycin.
(d) It may present as a hyperlucent lung.
(e) Recurrence in the irradiated field may be suggested by absence of ectatic bronchi on CT.

Q18 Are the following statements regarding AIDS-related lymphoma true or false?

(a) It occurs in the early stage of the disease.
(b) It is the commonest pulmonary neoplasm in patients with AIDS.
(c) It may present with a chest wall mass.

(d) Mediastinal adenopathy is present in 90%.
(e) The prognosis is poor.

Q19 Are the following statements true or false? In thoracic trauma:

(a) rib fractures are found in 50% of cases of significant pulmonary trauma.
(b) the ninth, tenth and eleventh ribs are the most commonly fractured.
(c) rib fractures are more common on the right.
(d) flail chest occurs when two fractures happen in the same rib.
(e) extrapleural haematomas are best seen on an oblique view.

Q20 Are the following statements regarding cystic fibrosis true or false?

(a) It is due to a defective gene on chromosome 7.
(b) The radiological findings have a predilection for the apical and posterior segments of the upper lobes.
(c) The cause of death is massive mucus plugging in 5% of cases.
(d) It is associated with hypoplasia of the frontal sinuses.
(e) It has a median survival of 28 years.

Q21 Are the following statements regarding the venous anatomy of the chest true or false?

(a) The accessory hemiazygos system drains into the hemiazygos system at T12.
(b) The coronary sinus opens into the left atrium.
(c) The internal thoracic (mammary) veins drain into the superior aspect of the brachiocephalic veins.
(d) The great cardiac vein ascends in the anterior interventricular groove.
(e) The bronchial veins drain on the right into the azygos system and on the left into the hemiazygos system.

The following are recognised pulmonary complications of trauma. True or false?

(a) Pulmonary arteriovenous fistula.
(b) Diaphragmatic rupture.
(c) Chylous effusion.
(d) Mirizzi's syndrome.
(e) Tracheal fracture.

 Are the following statements true or false? In percutaneous lung biopsies:

(a) the likelihood of tumour dissemination is greater with cutting needles.
(b) air embolism may occur.
(c) mediastinal emphysema is a common complication.
(d) the incidence of pneumothorax is less than 5%.
(e) compressed collagen plugs along the needle track may reduce the incidence of pneumothorax.

 Are the following statements regarding mesothelioma true or false?

(a) It is always malignant.
(b) It may be assessed with Butchart staging.
(c) Pleural plaques are present in 90%.
(d) It usually destroys the underlying rib.
(e) It may simulate fibrothorax.

 Are the following statements regarding thymic cysts true or false?

(a) They typically occur in the posterior mediastinum.
(b) They are associated with human immunodeficiency virus (HIV).
(c) They are linked with myasthenia gravis.
(d) They are hyperechoic on US.
(e) Fifty per cent are calcified.

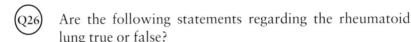

Q26 Are the following statements regarding the rheumatoid lung true or false?

(a) Interstitial fibrosis is the commonest thoracic manifestation.
(b) Caplan's syndrome occurs in malt workers.
(c) Bronchiectasis is a complication.
(d) Pulmonary arterial involvement does not occur.
(e) Centrilobular nodules have been described.

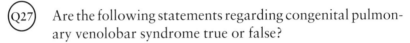

Q27 Are the following statements regarding congenital pulmonary venolobar syndrome true or false?

(a) The pulmonary artery is absent in 10–20%.
(b) It is commoner on the left side.
(c) A scimitar vein is seen in 10–20%.
(d) It is associated with congenital heart disease in 25–50%.
(e) Rib notching is not seen.

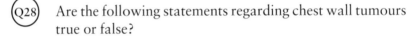

Q28 Are the following statements regarding chest wall tumours true or false?

(a) Glomus tumours are associated with calcification on plain film.
(b) Cavernous haemangiomas may demonstrate fluid levels.
(c) Leiomyosarcoma is associated with AIDS.
(d) Chronic lymphoedema predisposes to angiosarcoma.
(e) All chondrosarcomas arise from previous benign tumours.

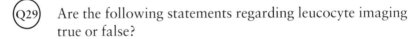

Q29 Are the following statements regarding leucocyte imaging true or false?

(a) Indium-111 may be used.
(b) The maximum activity is at four hours.
(c) Diffuse pulmonary uptake is always normal.
(d) Focal uptake may be seen in cystic fibrosis.
(e) Technetium-99 may also be used as an agent.

The following are thoracic complications of drug abuse. True or false?

(a) Upper lobe emphysema.
(b) Pulmonary amyloidosis.
(c) Lipoma.
(d) Aortic rupture.
(e) Pulmonary hypertension.

Answers

(A1) (a) False.
    (b) True.
    (c) False.
    (d) True.
    (e) False.

Severe acute respiratory distress syndrome is caused by SARS-associated coronavirus (SARS-CoV). The diagnosis is currently based on a combination of clinical information and imaging features. CXR and high-resolution CT (HRCT) are the main imaging modalities to be used. 22% of patients have a normal CXR at presentation. Unifocal consolidation is the most common finding at presentation. Other findings on plain film include: air-space opacification, lower and peripheral lung involvement and right lung more commonly affected than left lung. Radiological features on HRCT include: ground-glass opacification with or without consolidation, lower lobe, peripheral and subpleural predilection, commonly multifocal or bilateral involvement and thickening of the inter and intralobular septa with ground-glass opacification (crazy paving appearance). Cavitation, calcification, lymphadenopathy or pleural effusions are not usually encountered. HRCT is used as an adjunct to CXR in those patients who have a normal plain film but for whom a high index of clinical suspicion remains.

(A2) (a) True.
    (b) True.

(c) False.
(d) True.
(e) True.

Alveolar cell carcinoma accounts for 1–6% of lung cancers. There are several risk factors including previous fibrosis, heavy cigarette smoking and exogenous lipoid pneumonia. These cancers typically occur peripherally with marked tracheobronchial dissemination. They are unifocal in 60–90%, in the form of increased ground-glass attenuation and/or a focal mass. Alveolar cells are the second commonest cell type to cause cavitation. The CT angiogram sign signifies low attenuation consolidation that does not obscure vessels (seen in the mucin-producing type of alveolar cell carcinoma).

   (a) True.
(b) False.
(c) False:
(d) True.
(e) False.

Most cases of CFA (or usual interstitial pneumonia, UIP) are idiopathic. Others cases are familial, drug related or associated with connective tissue diseases such as rheumatoid arthritis. NSIP may be due to connective tissue diseases, infection, or toxic inhalation. LCH is severely accelerated by cigarette smoking.

   (a) True.
(b) True.
(c) True.
(d) True.
(e) True.

A linear probe (5–7.5 MHz) is ideal for sonographic examination of the chest. The diagnosis of rib fractures is made twice as frequently on US than on plain film. A pneumothorax may be confirmed on US by a number of features: absence of breath-related movement of the visceral pleura ('gliding sign') and markedly increased reverberation artefacts. However, if the pneumothorax is extensive, the artefacts are occasionally absent. Low resistance tumour flow signifies abnormal neovascularisation. On US, a pulmonary infarct is typically 1–2 cm smaller than the perfusion defect on angiography or scintigraphy. In a few cases, the thrombosed vessel can be seen (vessel sign).

 (a) False.
   (b) True.
   (c) False.
   (d) True.
   (e) True.

MRI does not necessarily require contrast for the diagnosis of pulmonary thromboembolism. Its multiplanar capability, ability to assess flow and the potential source of thrombus (e.g. pelvic veins) all add to its advantages, although it is not widely available. A false-positive diagnosis may also be caused by hilar nodes, partial opacification of the vessels and the partial voluming effect. Subsegmental thrombi may be visualised with 2 mm collimation. The risk of mortality from pulmonary angiography is less than 1%, however, the subgroup of patients who have pulmonary hypertension are at increased risk.

 (a) False.
   (b) True.
   (c) True.
   (d) True.
   (e) True.

Lung torsion typically occurs in the acute phase. Diseases that have recurred in the transplanted lung include: diffuse panbronchiolitis, alveolar proteinosis, giant cell pneumonia, desquamative interstitial pneumonia (DIP) and lymphangioleiomyomatosis.

 (a) False.
   (b) True.
   (c) True.
   (d) True.
   (e) True.

Left-sided atrial myxomas are the commonest primary cardiac tumours. Patients with tuberous sclerosis should be investigated for cardiac rhabdomyomas. Rhabdomyomas in newborns often regress spontaneously. Cardiac fibromas appear as solitary calcified/cystic lesions in the ventricular myocardium.

 (a) True.
(b) True.
(c) False.
(d) True.
(e) False.

 (a) True.
(b) True.
(c) False.
(d) True.
(e) False.

Multiple conditions result in this appearance on V/Q scans including acute and chronic thromboembolism, bronchogenic carcinoma, previous radiotherapy, vasculitis, hypoplasia of the pulmonary artery and hilar adenopathy.

 (a) False.
(b) False.
(c) True.
(d) True.
(e) False.

Pericardial defects are due to premature atrophy of the left cardinal vein, which then fails to nourish the developing pleuropericardial membrane. It is three times more common in men and occurs in all age groups. It is partially absent in 91%, being much more common on the left. Pericardial defects are associated with a variety of disorders, such as bronchogenic cysts (30%), ventricular septal defects (VSD), patent ductus arteriosus (PDA), mitral stenosis, diaphragmatic hernia and pulmonary sequestration. They may present with chest pain or may, in fact, be asymptomatic. Depending on the size of the defects, they may result in herniation of cardiac structures or lung, even leading to laevoposition of the heart. They generally require surgical intervention.

(a) False.
(b) True.
(c) True.
(d) False.
(e) True.

Thallium-201 chloride, technetium-99m sestamibi/tetrofosmin/ teboroxime are all nuclear medicine agents commonly used in the diagnosis of ischaemic heart disease. The myocardial uptake and blood clearance of all of these agents is very rapid, most having 5% activity remaining at 5–10 minutes post injection. The reverse distribution pattern is defined as the development of a new perfusion defect on thallium-201 images compared with the immediate post-stress images. It may occur with coronary artery disease, however, it is not specific or sensitive and may occur in other conditions such as post-coronary artery surgery, cardiac transplantation, Wolff–Parkinson–White syndrome and Kawasaki's disease. Quantitative analysis of myocardial imaging may be obtained from both planar imaging (histogram) and via single-photon emission computed tomography (SPECT) (bull's eye display).

 (a) True.
(b) False.
(c) True.
(d) False.
(e) True.

Cryptogenic organising pneumonia (COP), also termed BOOP (bronchiolitis obliterans with organising pneumonia), typically occurs in the 40–70-years age group. It has a wide variety of causes including post-obstructive pneumonia, acute respiratory distress syndrome (ARDS), lung carcinoma, extrinsic allergic alveolitis (EAA), collagen vascular disease, drug toxicity, and it may be idiopathic. Granulation tissue polyps fill the alveolar ducts and respiratory bronchioles with a varying degree of infiltration of the interstitium. It occurs in a mid- and lower-zone distribution, in the subpleural and peribronchiolar regions. HRCT features include patchy airspace consolidation (80%), ground-glass change (60%), centrilobular nodules (30–50%), air bronchograms, pleural effusions and adenopathy. Many patients improve with corticosteroid therapy.

 A13
(a) True.
(b) True.
(c) True.
(d) False.
(e) True.

Lipoid pneumonia (due to oil inhalation) usually causes consolidation in the lower lobes, which is of fat density on CT. Alveolar proteinosis is the only pure alveolar disease in which excess surfactant accumulates. Pulmonary contusion typically causes acute alveolar infiltrate.

 A14
(a) True.
(b) True.
(c) True.
(d) True.
(e) True.

Lymphoid interstitial pneumonia is a benign disorder characterised by diffuse infiltration of small mature lymphocytes and plasma cells. Other associated conditions include systemic lupus erythematosus, myasthenia gravis, pernicious anaemia, and Sjögren's syndrome. It is bilateral and involves all zones, and may be progressive in a third of cases.

 A15
(a) True.
(b) True.
(c) False.
(d) True.
(e) False.

The interstitial septa of the normal lung are not normally visible on plain CXR, apart from in very thin patients. For practical purposes, they are only visible when they become thickened. Deep septal lines (Kerley A) are up to 4 cm in length and radiate from the central portions of the lungs. However, they do not reach the pleura and are most obvious in the mid and upper zones. Kerley B lines are usually less than 1 cm in length and parallel each other at right angles to the pleura, generally occurring in a more peripheral position.

 (a) False.
(b) False.
(c) True.
(d) True.
(e) True.

The transverse sinus lies posterior to the ascending aorta and the pulmonary trunk, above the left atrium. The oblique sinus lies behind the left atrium and anterior to the oesophagus and has no direct connection with the superior pericardial recess. A right-sided aortic arch with mirror branch imaging has a 98% association with cyanotic congenital heart disease. The right atrium enlarges in a posterior direction.

 (a) False.
(b) False.
(c) True.
(d) True.
(e) True.

Radiographic changes are not necessarily associated with symptoms. They are most extensive at three to four months post radiation. Radiation-enhancing drugs such as bleomycin, adriamycin D, cyclophosphamide and vincristine may increase the degree of damage and shorten the time of onset. Apart from consolidation, this condition may present as a hyperlucency, pneumothorax, pleural effusions and calcified lymph nodes. Recurrence in treated areas may manifest as a change in stable contours of radiation fibrosis and failure of contraction of radiation pneumonitis four months after cessation of treatment.

 (a) False.
(b) False.
(c) True.
(d) False.
(e) True.

AIDS-related lymphoma is usually seen when the CD4 count is below 100–500 cells/mm^3. Kaposi's sarcoma is the commonest neoplasm in this cohort. Only 20–25% have mediastinal adenopathy, and the prognosis is generally very poor, with a median survival of five to seven months.

 (a) True.
(b) False.
(c) False.
(d) True.
(e) True.

The sixth, seventh and eighth ribs are the most commonly fractured.

 (a) True.
(b) True.
(c) False.
(d) True.
(e) True.

Cystic fibrosis is a genetically inherited autosomal recessive disorder. It is due to a mutation on the long arm of chromosome 7 (transmembrane conductance regulator gene). Pulmonary complications are the commonest cause of death, with massive mucus plugging as the cause in 95%. The median survival is 28 years, with 78% of patients suffering from cardiorespiratory disease. Thoracic features include a predilection for the apical and posterior segments of the upper lobes, mucus plugging, subsegmental atelectasis, bronchiectasis, hyperinflation, hilar adenopathy, recurrent pneumonitis, pulmonary hypertension and allergic bronchopulmonary aspergillosis. Extrathoracic features include: gastrointestinal (meconium plug syndrome, meconium ileus, fibrosing colonopathy, rectal prolapse, appendicitis, jejunisation of the colon, thickened nodular duodenal folds), hepatic (steatosis, biliary cirrhosis and portal hypertension), pancreatic (acute and chronic pancreatitis, fatty replacement and calcification, pancreatic cystosis, i.e. microscopic cyst formation replacing the body of the pancreas) and ENT manifestations (sinusitis, hypoplasia of the frontal sinuses).

(a) False.
(b) False.
(c) False.
(d) True.
(e) True.

The accessory hemiazygos and hemiazygos systems drain into the azygos system at T8, either separately or via a common trunk. The accessory hemiazygos system receives the fourth to eighth posterior intercostal veins; the hemiazygos system receives the lowermost four intercostal veins, the left ascending lumbar, the mediastinal and the oesophageal veins.

The coronary sinus opens into the posterior wall of the right atrium and lies in the posterior interventricular groove. The great cardiac vein ascends in the anterior interventricular groove, the middle cardiac vein ascends in the posterior interventricular groove. The internal thoracic veins drain into the inferior aspect of both brachiocephalic veins. The bronchial arteries arise directly from the aorta in 90% of cases – one on the right and one on the left being the commonest configuration. The right bronchial vein typically drains into the azygos system and the left drains into the hemi-azygos system.

 (a) True.
(b) True.
(c) True.
(d) False.
(e) True.

Chylous effusion or chylothorax occurs due to disruption of the thoracic duct or its branches as they ascend in the chest. It may be due to closed or open chest trauma, and it may take one to two weeks after the trauma to manifest. Mirizzi's syndrome describes obstruction of the common hepatic duct by an inflamed gall-bladder.

 (a) True.
(b) True.
(c) False.

(d) False.
(e) True.

The incidence of pneumothorax is 10–40% on CT. Mediastinal emphysema is rare.

 A24   (a) False.
(b) True.
(c) False.
(d) False.
(e) True.

Benign mesothelioma is a recognised entity and accounts for less than 5% of cases. Pleural plaques are present in 50%.

 A25   (a) False.
(b) True.
(c) False.
(d) False.
(e) False.

Thymic cysts may be congenital or acquired. Thymomas are linked with myasthenia gravis. The cysts are anechoic on US, calcification being a rare feature. Histologically, they are thin-walled cysts with thymic tissue and are generally 0–10 hounsfield units (HU) on CT.

 A26   (a) False.
(b) False.
(c) True.
(d) False.
(e) True.

Pleural disease is the commonest manifestation (pleural effusion, pericarditis). Caplan's syndrome occurs in patients with both rheumatoid lung and coal worker's pneumoconiosis. Pulmonary arteritis has been described. Follicular bronchiolitis may occur (centrilobular nodules with ground-glass change).

 A27   (a) True.
(b) False.
(c) False.

(d) True.
(e) False.

Congenital pulmonary venolobar syndrome is slightly commoner on the right and in females. A scimitar vein (partial anomalous pulmonary venous drainage) is seen in 80–90%. Rib notching is seen due to collateral formation.

  (a) False.
(b) True.
(c) True.
(d) True.
(e) False.

Glomus tumours are rare in adulthood; they are associated with bone erosion rather than calcification (cavernous haemangiomas). Leiomyosarcomas account for less than 5% of soft-tissue sarcomas, occurring typically in the 50–70-years age group. In children and adolescents, leiomyosarcomas are associated with AIDS and other immunosuppressive disorders. Previous irradiation and chemical exposure are also risk factors in the development of angiosarcoma. Chondrosarcomas may also arise *de novo*.

  (a) True.
(b) False.
(c) False.
(d) True.
(e) True.

The maximum activity is within a few minutes, with complete washout typically at four hours. Diffuse pulmonary uptake after four hours is abnormal and may be found in a variety of conditions such as ARDS, drug-induced toxicity, opportunistic infections, radiation pneumonitis and sepsis. Causes of focal uptake include atelectasis, pulmonary embolism, congestive cardiac failure (CCF) and infection.

  (a) True.
(b) True.
(c) False.

(d) True.
(e) True.

Intravenous (IV) injection of oral medication is associated with upper lobe emphysema; IV methylphenidate is a causative agent of lower lobe emphysema. Talcosis may lead to formation of pulmonary amyloidosis. Cocaine is associated with aortic dissection and rupture.

Section 2

Cardiovascular

Q1 Are the following statements regarding an aberrant left pulmonary artery true or false?

(a) The left pulmonary artery passes between the trachea and oesophagus.
(b) The condition typically presents in adulthood.
(c) The condition is frequently associated with patent ductus arteriosus (PDA).
(d) Obstructive emphysema of the right and left lower lobes is typical.
(e) The trachea narrows in a cephalad direction.

Q2 Are the following statements regarding thoracic aortic aneurysms true or false?

(a) Curvilinear calcification is seen in less than 50% of cases.
(b) The lung is typically consolidated adjacent to an area of aneurysmal dilatation.
(c) Most aneurysms rupture at a diameter of 6–7 cm.
(d) Angiography may demonstrate normal aortic diameter even with an aneurysm present.
(e) Rupture demonstrates leak of high attenuation fluid.

Q3 Are the following statements regarding the aortic isthmus true or false?

(a) The aortic isthmus is sited proximal to the ductus arteriosus.
(b) The aortic isthmus should not be apparent after three months of age.

21

(c) A ductus diverticulum is present on the lateral aspect of the aortic isthmus.

(d) An aortic spindle is seen just proximal to the aortic isthmus.

(e) It is a common site for traumatic aortic rupture.

Q4 Are the following statements regarding aortic dissections true or false?

(a) Those affecting the abdominal aorta usually originate in the thoracic aorta.

(b) They are associated with aortic coarctation.

(c) Mesenteric ischaemia in type B dissection is an indication for surgery.

(d) The false lumen is usually posterolaterally placed in the ascending aorta.

(e) The false lumen is usually larger than the true lumen.

Q5 Are the following statements regarding abdominal aortic aneurysms true or false?

(a) Approximately 50% are suprarenal.

(b) They are correlated with popliteal artery aneurysms.

(c) Mycotic aneurysms are typically fusiform and concentric.

(d) Aortocaval fistula may lead to congestive heart failure.

(e) A peripheral high attenuation intramural crescent is a sign of impending rupture.

Q6 Are the following statements regarding Takayasu's arteritis true or false?

(a) The pulmonary arteries are involved in less than 30% of cases.

(b) Stenosis is commoner in the abdominal than the thoracic aorta.

(c) Enhancement of aortic wall with contrast is a recognised feature.

(d) Saccular aneurysms are seen.

(e) Forty per cent of patients are over 30 years of age.

Q7 Are the following statements regarding the splenic artery true or false?

(a) It gives off the short gastric arteries.

(b) It gives off the pancreatica magna artery in the head of the pancreas.

(c) It reaches the spleen via the gastrosplenic ligament.

(d) It commonly calcifies to give a 'dragon's tail' appearance.

(e) It usually gives off the right gastric artery.

Q8 Are the following statements regarding CO_2 angiography true or false?

(a) The CO_2 cylinder can be connected directly to the patient via a safety valve.

(b) CO_2 can be used for brachial arteriography.

(c) CO_2 venography is contraindicated in patients with right-to-left cardiac shunts.

(d) Up to 100 ml can be used per minute.

(e) CO_2 angiography tends to overestimate vessel size.

Q9 Are the following statements regarding the magnetic resonance angiography (MRA) technique true or false?

(a) Time of flight (TOF) angiography uses a gradient echo sequence in which flowing blood appears bright.

(b) Phase contrast imaging is usually faster than TOF.

(c) Echo planar imaging is often helpful in contrast-enhanced MRA.

(d) Phase contrast imaging gives quantitative data on flow.

(e) TOF can be used to measure in-plane flow.

Q10 Are the following statements regarding aortic arch angiography true or false?

(a) The arch and great vessels are best demonstrated on the left anterior oblique view.
(b) An injection volume of 20 ml is usually sufficient.
(c) A frame rate of two to four frames per second is usually required.
(d) A 7 French or larger catheter should be used.
(e) The commonest site of injury in traumatic aortic rupture is at the aortic root.

Q11 Are the following statements regarding the hepatic vascular supply true or false?

(a) Aberrant arterial supply is present in up to 40% of patients.
(b) The left hepatic artery arises from the left gastric artery in 10–20% of patients.
(c) The entire hepatic artery supply arises from the superior mesenteric artery (SMA) in 0.2% of patients.
(d) Non-tumour-related perfusion defects are seen in 30% of CT-arterioportograms.
(e) The portal vein contributes 25–30% of blood flow to the liver.

Q12 Are the following statements regarding cardiac atrial septal defects (ASD) true or false?

(a) The ostium primum type is more common than ostium secundum.
(b) ASD with ostium primum is associated with the Holt–Oram syndrome.
(c) ASD often presents with pulmonary hypertension.
(d) The left atrium and ventricle are typically enlarged.
(e) The heart tends to rotate anticlockwise.

Q13 Are the following statements regarding mesenteric angiography for gastrointestinal bleeding true or false?

(a) Angiography is more sensitive than nuclear medicine red cell scan.
(b) The vitelline artery supplying a Meckel's diverticulum extends beyond the mesentery.
(c) Late venous filling is a sign of angiodysplasia.
(d) Diverticular bleeding is usually venous.
(e) If possible, the SMA is cannulated first in angiography for colonic bleeding.

 Q14 The following are recognised causes of cardiomegaly. True or false?

(a) Uhl's disease.
(b) Fallot's tetralogy.
(c) Tricuspid atresia.
(d) Ebstein's anomaly.
(e) Pulmonary atresia.

 Q15 Are the following statements regarding the pericardium true or false?

(a) Cardiac surgery is a recognised cause of constrictive pericarditis.
(b) Of patients with constrictive pericarditis 30% have pericardial calcification.
(c) A pericardial effusion of 150 ml is usually detectable on plain film.
(d) Partial absence of the pericardium is commoner than total absence.
(e) Pericardial cysts are commonest in the middle mediastinum.

 Q16 Are the following statements regarding asplenia true or false?

(a) Both bronchi are hyparterial.
(b) There is an association with ASD.

(c)   Transposition of the great arteries (TGA) is associated with asplenia in 70% of cases.

(d)   Situs inversus or ambiguus is associated with asplenia.

(e)   Asplenia has a worse prognosis than polysplenia.

 Q17   Are the following statements regarding thoracic outlet syndrome true or false?

(a)   The commonest congenital cause is an anomalous first rib.

(b)   Compression by scalenus posterior is a recognised cause.

(c)   Angiography may demonstrate post-stenotic dilatation of the subclavian artery.

(d)   The commonest acquired cause is a fracture of the clavicle or first rib.

(e)   Duplex ultrasound of the subclavian artery with the patient's neck flexed is a sensitive test.

 Q18   Are the following statements regarding priapism true or false?

(a)   The commonest cause is unregulated arterial flow into the corpora cavernosa.

(b)   The veno-occlusive form is characterised by ischaemia within the penis.

(c)   The arterial form is characterised by a painful erection.

(d)   Arterial inflow is decreased in the veno-occlusive form.

(e)   Impotence subsequently occurs in >40% of cases.

 Q19   Are the following statements regarding renal artery stenosis (RAS) true or false?

(a)   RAS is present in about 40% of patients with malignant hypertension.

(b)   A size disparity of 1 cm warrants investigation.

(c)   On intravenous urogram, notching of the proximal ureter is supportive evidence.

(d) A post-stenotic dilatation is 70–85% predictive of flow-limiting stenosis.

(e) Duplex ultrasound is a highly sensitive test.

Q20 Are the following statements regarding RAS due to fibromuscular dysplasia (FMD) true or false?

(a) It is three times commoner in females.

(b) The proximal renal artery is almost always spared.

(c) There is a recognised association with FMD in the carotid or mesenteric artery.

(d) It is bilateral in a third of cases.

(e) It is commoner on the right side.

Q21 Are the following statements regarding varicocele true or false?

(a) There is a recognised association with infertility.

(b) It is commoner on the right side alone than bilaterally.

(c) Varicocele present only with Valsalva's manoeuvre is associated with normal sperm quality.

(d) The commonest congenital cause is an incompetent or absent valve of the inferior vena cava or left gonadal vein.

(e) Occlusion of the testicular vein is a recognised treatment.

Q22 Are the following statements regarding CT coronary angiography true or false?

(a) Imaging is performed during systole.

(b) The proportion of time spent in systole increases with heart rate.

(c) Glyceryl trinitrate (GTN) may be used to aid visualisation of the coronary arteries.

(d) Heart rate tends to decrease after prolonged breath holding.

(e) Motion artefact is greater for the right coronary artery (RCA) than for the left anterior descending (LAD) artery.

Q23 Are the following statements regarding coronary artery anatomy true or false?

(a) The main vessels have a diameter of 0.5–2 mm at their origin.

(b) Usually the left coronary artery (LCA) gives rise to the posterior descending artery.

(c) The LCA is constant in diameter.

(d) The RCA may trifurcate, giving rise to the ramus intermedius artery.

(e) The acute marginal artery supplies part of the left ventricle.

 Q24 Are the following statements regarding coronary artery calcification true or false?

(a) The calcified lesion represents 40–70% of the total atheroma burden in the vessel.

(b) It is well detected by coronary angiography.

(c) It is an independent risk factor for coronary artery thrombosis.

(d) Lack of coronary artery calcification excludes the presence of atheroma.

(e) Agatston scoring takes into account the attenuation of the calcified lesion as well as the size.

 Q25 Are the following statements regarding deep vein thrombosis (DVT) true or false?

(a) DVT is commoner in the right leg than the left.

(b) Tamoxifen is a risk factor.

(c) Bilateral negative venograms may sometimes be seen with proved pulmonary emboli.

(d) Venous diameter twice that of the artery suggests old established clot.

(e) Venograms are falsely negative in approximately 10% of cases.

Are the following statements regarding CT pulmonary angiography (CTPA) for pulmonary embolic disease true or false?

(a) CTPA is as sensitive as catheter angiography down to the fifth division of the pulmonary artery.
(b) Sensitivity is greatest in the middle and lingular lobes.
(c) Interobserver agreement for catheter angiography is greater than 90%.
(d) Approximately 70% of ventilation/perfusion (V/Q) scans are indeterminate.
(e) Abrupt vessel cut-off is a sign of acute pulmonary embolism.

 Are the following statements regarding carotid artery stenosis and its assessment true or false?

(a) A reduction in vessel diameter of 50% will normally limit flow.
(b) The commonest site affected is the carotid siphon.
(c) Endarterectomy of >70% stenosis reduces ipsilateral stroke at two years by 70%.
(d) Calcifications up to 2 cm do not hinder assessment by duplex ultrasound.
(e) A peak systolic velocity of 100 cm/s is normal.

 Are the following statements regarding the internal carotid artery (ICA) true or false?

(a) The cervical segment of the ICA has no branches.
(b) The cavernous segment exits laterally to the anterior clinoid process.
(c) The ICA ascends medially to the external carotid artery.
(d) The ophthalmic artery arises from the supraclinoid segment.
(e) The anterior choroidal artery arises proximally to the posterior communicating artery.

Are the following statements regarding MRA of the carotid artery true or false?

(a) MRA is more sensitive than duplex ultrasound for detecting high-grade (>70%) stenoses.
(b) Three-dimensional TOF sequences may underestimate stenosis.
(c) Phase contrast MRA allows assessment of direction of flow.
(d) Phase contrast MRA is more susceptible than TOF imaging to signal dropout from turbulent flow.
(e) Presence of a normal flow void excludes a significant stenosis.

 Are the following statements regarding the renal vessels true or false?

(a) Accessory renal vessels are commoner in horseshoe kidneys.
(b) Accessory renal arteries are seen in 2% of patients.
(c) The right renal vein is usually longer than the left.
(d) The renal vein lies posterior to the renal artery.
(e) The main renal artery has branches passing anterior and posterior to the renal pelvis.

Answers

 (a) True.
(b) False.
(c) True.
(d) False.
(e) False.

Aberrant left pulmonary artery usually presents in childhood. It is due to a developmental failure of the left sixth aortic arch resulting in the formation of a collateral vessel from the right pulmonary artery to supply the left lung. The resulting vessel may appear as a soft-tissue mass between the trachea and oesophagus, causing narrowing of the trachea in a caudal direction and obstructive emphysema or atelectasis of the right and left upper lobes. The anomaly is frequently associated with congenital heart diseases such as patent ductus arteriosus and atrial septal defect.

 A2
- (a) False.
- (b) True.
- (c) False.
- (d) True.
- (e) True.

Thoracic aortic aneurysms are associated with peripheral curvilinear calcification in approximately 75% of cases. An area of consolidated lung is often seen adjacent to the aneurysm, which may occasionally cause diagnostic confusion. Most aneurysms rupture at a diameter of 10 cm (in contrast with abdominal aortic aneurysms). Angiography may appear normal due to mural thrombus masking the extent of the aneurysm. Leaks are normally high attenuation.

 A3
- (a) True.
- (b) True.
- (c) False.
- (d) False.
- (e) True.

An aortic isthmus is an aortic narrowing distal to the left subclavian artery and proximal to the ductus arteriosus that disappears by two months of age due to decreased flow in the ductus and increased flow through the narrowed segment. A ductus diverticulum presents as a smooth, symmetrical (or occasionally asymmetrical) bulge on the anteromedial aspect of the aortic isthmus. An aortic spindle is a normal variant placed below the isthmus. Ninety-five per cent of aortic ruptures occur at the isthmus since the aorta is relatively fixed here.

 A4
- (a) True.
- (b) True.
- (c) True.

(d) False.
(e) True.

Aortic dissections almost exclusively arise in the thoracic aorta and may involve the abdominal aorta by extension. They are associated with aortic coarctation and bicuspid aortic valve. Although type B is usually treated medically, indications for surgery are: renal, mesenteric or extremity ischaemia; aneurysmal enlargement of false lumen; or rupture. The false lumen is usually anterolaterally placed in the ascending aorta and posterolateral in the descending aorta. The false lumen is usually larger than the true lumen.

 (a) False.
(b) True.
(c) False.
(d) True.
(e) True.

Ninety per cent of abdominal aortic aneurysms are infrarenal; they are correlated with hypertension and popliteal artery aneurysms. Mycotic aneurysms are typically saccular and eccentric and are commoner in sepsis, bacterial endocarditis and after arterial trauma. Aortocaval fistula may lead to rapidly progressive heart failure. Acute intramural haematoma is indicated by a peripheral high attenuation crescent and is serious as it is a sign of impending rupture.

 (a) False.
(b) False.
(c) True.
(d) True.
(e) False.

Ninety per cent of patients with Takayasu's arteritis are 30 years old or less (unlike other arteritides). Acutely, arterial wall thickening and contrast enhancement are seen, with full-thickness calcification in chronic disease. Aortic stenosis (commoner in the thoracic aorta) or dilatation may be seen, with occasional saccular aneurysm formation. The pulmonary arteries are involved in 50%

of cases, with pruning of peripheral vessels and dilatation of the pulmonary trunk.

 (a) True.
(b) False.
(c) True.
(d) True.
(e) False.

The splenic artery gives off the pancreatica magna artery in the tail of the pancreas. It usually gives off the left gastric artery.

 (a) False.
(b) False.
(c) True.
(d) False.
(e) False.

CO_2 angiography is a useful alternative to iodinated contrast in cases where there is concern about contrast reaction or nephrotoxicity. CO_2 is drawn up into a 50 ml or 60 ml syringe and then injected – the CO_2 cylinder should never be connected directly to the patient. CO_2 arteriography should not be performed above the diaphragm nor should CO_2 venography be performed in patients with right-to-left cardiac shunts because of the risk of cerebral embolism. Up to 100 ml can be used every two minutes. Because CO_2 does not fill the dependent parts of the blood vessels it tends to underestimate vessel size.

 (a) True.
(b) False.
(c) True.
(d) True.
(e) False.

Phase contrast imaging is slower than TOF, which is slower than contrast-enhanced MRA. Echo planar imaging is helpful in all types of MRA. Phase contrast imaging gives quantitative data on flow as opposed to TOF and contrast-enhanced. TOF cannot be used to measure in-plane flow.

(a) False.
(b) False.
(c) True.
(d) False.
(e) False.

The arch and origin of the branch vessels are best demonstrated on a 30-degree or occasionally 60-degree right anterior oblique view. In order to fill and visualise the vessels an injection volume of approximately 50 ml and frame rate of two to four frames per second are required. A 4 or 5-french pigtail catheter is sufficient. The commonest site of injury in traumatic aortic rupture is where the aorta is fixed at the ligamentum arteriosum.

 (a) True.
(b) True.
(c) False.
(d) False.
(e) False.

The commonest hepatic vascular supply anomalies are the right hepatic artery originating from SMA and left hepatic artery originating from left gastric artery (each in approximately 20% of patients). In 2% of patients, the entire hepatic arterial supply is from the SMA. Non-tumour-related perfusion defects are seen in 70% of CT-arterioportograms, most commonly at the junction of segments 4A and 4B. The portal vein contributes 70–75% of blood flow to the liver.

 (a) False.
(b) False.
(c) True.
(d) False.
(e) False.

ASD is the commonest congenital cardiac anomaly: ostium primum is rarer and more complicated than ostium secundum and is associated with Down's syndrome (ostium secundum is associated with Holt–Oram syndrome). ASD is often asymptomatic until adulthood, commonly presenting with pulmonary hypertension. The right atrium and ventricle are usually enlarged and are associated with clockwise rotation.

 A13
    (a) False.
    (b) True.
    (c) False.
    (d) True.
    (e) False.

Nuclear medicine red cell scan is more sensitive than angiography, being able to detect bleeding rates of 0.1 ml/min versus 1 ml/min. The vitelline artery supplying a Meckel's diverticulum can be recognised by the following features: it extends beyond the mesentery, has no side branches and ends in a corkscrew appearance. Angiodysplasia is characterised angiographically as a focal area of increased vascularity with dilated arterioles and a prominent early draining vein. Since diverticular bleeding is usually venous it may be difficult to demonstrate. Traditionally the inferior mesenteric artery is cannulated first since it is more difficult to appreciate once the bladder is full of contrast.

 A14
    (a) True.
    (b) False.
    (c) True.
    (d) True.
    (e) True.

Uhl's disease (total or focal absence of right ventricular myocardium), Ebstein's anomaly (congenital malformation characterised by apical displacement of the septal and posterior tricuspid valve leaflets, leading to atrialisation of the right ventricle), and tricuspid atresia lead to right atrial enlargement and cardiomegaly. Fallot's tetralogy causes a boot-shaped heart but typically without cardiomegaly. Pulmonary atresia is a recognised cause of cardiomegaly.

 A15
    (a) True.
    (b) False.
    (c) False.
    (d) True.
    (e) False.

Recognised causes of constrictive pericarditis include infection (especially tuberculosis), radiation and cardiac surgery. Among patients with constrictive pericarditis 90% have pericardial calcification, most commonly in the atrioventricular grooves. A pericardial effusion of 250 ml or more is usually required for detection on plain film. Partial absence of the pericardium is commoner than total absence, more commonly occurs on the left and, although usually asymptomatic, may present with cardiac strangulation. Pericardial cysts are commonest in the cardiophrenic angles.

 (a) False.
    (b) False.
    (c) True.
    (d) True.
    (e) True.

Asplenia (right isomerism) is associated with epiarterial bronchi, decreased pulmonary blood flow, bilateral minor fissures, a common atrium (as opposed to polysplenia which is associated with ASD), TGA and situs inversus or ambiguus (as is polysplenia). It has a worse prognosis than polysplenia.

 (a) False.
    (b) False.
    (c) True.
    (d) True.
    (e) False.

The commonest congenital cause is a cervical rib (up to 20% of symptomatic patients), with another common cause being compression by scalenus anterior (scalenus anticus syndrome). Duplex ultrasound is a sensitive test, with the patient's neck extended and shoulders back and with neck turned to either side.

 (a) False.
    (b) True.
    (c) False.
    (d) True.
    (e) True.

The commonest cause is veno-occlusive disease characterised by a painful erection, with decreased arterial and venous flow and ischaemia: predisposing risk factors are hypercoagulable states. The arterial form is rare, it occurs typically after perineal trauma and is characterised by a painless erection with unregulated arterial flow.

  (a) True.
(b) False.
(c) True.
(d) True.
(e) False.

Although only present in about 1% or less of all patients with hypertension, RAS is commoner in patients with difficult to control or malignant hypertension, and those with peripheral vascular disease. A right kidney 2 cm smaller than the left, or a left kidney 1.5 cm smaller than the right is supportive evidence. Notching of the proximal ureter is seen due to collateral vessels. Duplex ultrasound is relatively insensitive due to difficulties with visualisation of the entire artery, false tracings from collateral vessels, cardiac pulsation artefact and so on.

  (a) True.
(b) True.
(c) True.
(d) False.
(e) True.

RAS due to FMD spares the proximal renal artery in ~95% of cases. Rarely (in 1–2% of cases) there is associated disease of the carotid or mesenteric artery. It is bilateral in two-thirds of cases and four times commoner on the right side.

  (a) True.
(b) False.
(c) True.
(d) True.
(e) False.

Varicocele is thought to affect sperm quality for a number of reasons, particularly because it raises the temperature of the testicle. It is commoner bilaterally (16%) than on the right side alone (6%). Transcatheter occlusion of the gonadal vein is an established and effective treatment and is less invasive than surgery.

  (a) True.
(b) True.
(c) True.
(d) False.
(e) True.

Imaging is performed during systole and is easiest with a slow, regular heart rate. GTN has been used to vasodilate the coronary arteries and may aid visualisation although it may cause a counter-productive reflex tachycardia. Heart rate tends to increase after prolonged breath holding and so this is to be avoided. The LAD is least affected and the RCA most affected by motion artefact.

  (a) False.
(b) False.
(c) True.
(d) False.
(e) False.

The main vessels have a diameter of 2–4 mm at their origin, tapering to approximately 1 mm. In 85% of individuals the RCA gives rise to the posterior descending artery and posterior left ventricular branches (left dominant): in 8% both these arise from the left circumflex artery and in 7% the posterior descending artery arises from the RCA and the posterior left ventricular branches arise from the left circumflex artery.

  (a) False.
(b) False.
(c) True.
(d) False.
(e) True.

The calcified lesion itself represents approximately 20% of the atheromatous lesion. CT is much more sensitive than fluoroscopy for detecting coronary artery calcification. Lack of coronary artery calcification does not exclude non-calcified atheroma. Agatston scoring multiplies calcified lesion size by a factor related to its attenuation.

 (a) False.
(b) True.
(c) True.
(d) False.
(e) True.

DVT is about twice as common in the left leg; this is thought to be due to compression of the left common iliac vein by the left common iliac artery. Bilateral negative venograms may sometimes be seen with proved pulmonary emboli according to the 'big bang' theory that the clot from the leg may embolise en masse to the lungs. Thrombus typically expands the vein when fresh, later contracting. Venograms are approximately 90% sensitive and falsely positive in 5%.

 (a) True.
(b) False.
(c) False.
(d) True.
(e) True.

CTPA with multidetector CT is now able to detect subsegmental emboli with increasing sensitivity. Sensitivity is poorest for the middle and lingular lobes. There is only moderate interobserver agreement (60–70%) for emboli on catheter angiography. Abrupt vessel cut-off and intraluminal filling defects are specific signs of acute pulmonary embolism.

 (a) True.
(b) False.
(c) False.
(d) False.
(e) True.

The commonest site affected is the proximal internal carotid artery adjacent to the bifurcation. The NASCET trial showed a 17% reduction in ipsilateral stroke at two years after endarterectomy of >70% stenosis. Calcifications of up to 1 cm do not significantly hinder assessment by duplex ultrasound. The normal peak systolic velocity is up to 125 cm/s.

A28 (a) True.
(b) False.
(c) True.
(d) True.
(e) False.

The cavernous segment exits medially to the anterior clinoid process. The anterior choroidal artery arises distally to the posterior communicating artery and proximally to the bifurcation into middle and anterior cerebral arteries.

A29 (a) True.
(b) False.
(c) True.
(d) False.
(e) False.

MRA has been shown to be more sensitive than duplex ultrasound for detecting high grade (>70%) stenoses. Three-dimensional TOF sequences may overestimate stenosis. Phase contrast MRA is susceptible to signal loss due to turbulent flow causing intravoxel phase dispersion. A void may be seen even with significantly reduced flow.

A30 (a) True.
(b) False.
(c) False.
(d) False.
(e) True.

Accessory renal vessels represent fetal remnants and are seen in 20% of structurally normal kidneys and more commonly in horseshoe and ectopic kidneys. The left renal vein has to cross the aorta and is usually longer than the right, rendering it more suitable for organ donation. The renal vein is anterior to the renal artery, which usually has two branches passing anterior to and one branch passing posterior to the renal pelvis.

Section 3

Musculoskeletal (including trauma and soft tissues)

Q1 Are the following statements regarding radiography of the shoulder true or false?

(a) External rotation allows superior visualisation of a Hill–Sachs lesion.

(b) A type III acromion is associated with significantly more supraspinatus tears.

(c) The 40-degree posterior oblique view allows identification of the glenoid in profile.

(d) A 15-degree caudal tilt allows better assessment of the acromioclavicular joint.

(e) The axillary view is sufficient to assess for glenohumeral dislocation.

Q2 The following are causes of Erlenmeyer's flask deformity. True or false?

(a) Fibrous dysplasia.

(b) Thalassaemia.

(c) Acromegaly.

(d) Osteopetrosis.

(e) Schuermann's disease.

(Q3) The following conditions have malignant potential. True or false?

(a) Medullary bone infarct.
(b) Plexiform neurofibromatosis.
(c) Hyperphosphatasia.
(d) Previously irradiated bone.
(e) Osteopoikilosis.

(Q4) Are the following statements true or false?

(a) Tumoural calcinosis is an idiopathic disorder resulting in deposition of calcium within tendons and ligaments.
(b) Communicating hydrocephalus may result in posterior vertebral scalloping.
(c) Chondromyxoid fibroma is typically sclerotic.
(d) Periosteal desmoid tumours may be diagnosed only on bone biopsy.
(e) Telangiectatic osteosarcoma is a relatively indolent subtype of osteosarcoma.

(Q5) Are the following statements regarding trauma to the hip and pelvis true or false?

(a) The fat planes adjacent to the hip joint are sensitive indicators of the presence of joint fluid.
(b) Judet's views of the pelvis are equivalent to inlet views.
(c) Malgaigne's fractures of the pelvis are a combination of an ipsilateral sacroiliac and superior and inferior pubic rami fractures.
(d) The mortality in pelvic fractures is 1–5%.
(e) The Y vascular groove in the iliac bone requires investigation with angiography.

Are the following statements regarding magnetic resonance imaging (MRI) of joints true or false?

(a) The coronal plane is angled parallel to the volar surface of the radius.

(b) Short tan inversion recovery (STIR) sequences are unhelpful in the detection of occult fractures.

(c) Sagittal images of the knee are obtained perpendicular to a line drawn through both posterior femoral condyles.

(d) When imaging the shoulder, true sagittal sections are required.

(e) Signal-to-noise ratio is improved by three-dimensional volume acquisition.

Are the following statements regarding malignant fibrous histiocytoma (MFH) true or false?

(a) It is found most commonly in bone.

(b) It is sclerotic on plain film.

(c) In bone it occurs mostly in the metaphysis of the distal femur.

(d) It commonly occurs in children.

(e) It demonstrates increased uptake on bone scan.

The following locations are typical for the associated conditions. True or false?

(a) Implantation dermoid – terminal phalanx.

(b) Cortical desmoid – distal tibia.

(c) Chondroblastoma – epiphysis.

(d) Osteofibrous dysplasia – humerus.

(e) Intraosseous lipoma – calcaneum.

Are the following statements regarding lymphoma of bone true or false?

(a) Two-thirds of Hodgkin's disease deposits are solitary.

(b) The vertebral end plate is often destroyed.

(c)   In non-Hodgkin's lymphoma (NHL) bone involve-
      ment is commoner in children.
(d)   Burkitt's lymphoma typically affects the jaw.
(e)   Lymphoblastic NHL spreads to bone as a late feature.

(Q10)   Are the following statements true or false? Osteomalacia
        may be caused by:

(a)   dietary phosphorus deficiency.
(b)   biliary disease.
(c)   phenobarbitone.
(d)   in association with a tumour.
(e)   renal tubular acidosis.

(Q11)   Are the following statements true or false? Enthesopathy
        may occur with:

(a)   X-linked hypophosphataemia.
(b)   acromegaly.
(c)   Reiter's disease.
(d)   scurvy.
(e)   degenerative disease.

(Q12)   Are the following statements regarding hypervitamosis A
        true or false?

(a)   It causes metatarsal and ulnar hyperostosis.
(b)   It causes craniosynostosis.
(c)   It causes hair thickening.
(d)   It is associated with tendon calcification.
(e)   It causes delayed epiphyseal closure.

(Q13)   The following are recognised complications of fractures.
        True or false?

(a)   Aneurysmal bone cyst.
(b)   Osteoarthritis.
(c)   Sudeck's atrophy.
(d)   Lead arthropathy.
(e)   Myositis ossificans.

Q14 Stress fractures may occur in the following sites. True or false?

(a) Obturator ring.
(b) Upper cervical spinous processes.
(c) Sesamoid of metacarpals.
(d) Hamate.
(e) Trapezium.

Q15 Excessive bone callus occurs in the following conditions. True or false?

(a) Addison's disease.
(b) Neuropathic injury.
(c) Renal osteodystrophy.
(d) Hypercalcaemia.
(e) Multiple myeloma.

Q16 The differential diagnosis for bone sclerosis with a periosteal reaction includes the following conditions. True or false?

(a) Osteoid osteoma.
(b) Syphilis.
(c) Chondromyxoid fibroma.
(d) MFH.
(e) Lymphoma.

Q17 Are the following statements regarding fractures of the cervical spinal column true or false?

(a) All Jefferson's fractures are unstable.
(b) Forty per cent of C2 fractures are associated with head injuries.
(c) The commonest C2 fracture is a hangman's fracture.
(d) The 'ring' of C2 is always disrupted in odontoid peg fractures.
(e) Teardrop fractures of the vertebral bodies usually occur with spinal cord injuries.

Q18 Are the following statements regarding hand injuries true or false?

(a) Bennett's fractures are extra-articular.
(b) Fractures of the sesamoid bone of the thumb are usually vertical.
(c) The commonest carpometacarpal dislocation is at the fifth metacarpohamate joint.
(d) The commonest sites of fracture of the metacarpal base are the third and fourth fingers.
(e) Volar interphalangeal dislocation of the finger is commoner than the dorsal.

Q19 The following secondary signs on MRI help in the diagnosis of an anterior cruciate ligament (ACL) tear. True or false?

(a) Avulsion fracture of the posterior tibial eminence.
(b) Buckled posterior cruciate ligament (PCL).
(c) The entire length of the PCL is seen on coronal imaging.
(d) The lateral meniscus is 'uncovered'.
(e) Bone bruise in the anterior tibial plateau.

Q20 Are the following statements regarding soft tissues true or false?

(a) Elastofibroma typically occurs between the chest wall and the scapula.
(b) Muscle herniation most commonly occurs in the anterior compartment of the leg.
(c) Widespread soft-tissue calcification may be a manifestation of disseminated malignancy.
(d) Extra-abdominal desmoid tumour is locally aggressive.
(e) MRI may completely distinguish between lipoma and liposarcoma.

Q21 The following sites and nerves are correctly paired with respect to nerve entrapment syndromes. True or false?

(a) Median nerve – distal humerus.
(b) Axilla – radial nerve.
(c) Proximal fibula – posterior tibial nerve.
(d) Clavicle – suprascapular nerve.
(e) Anterior superior iliac spine – lateral femoral cutaneous nerve.

Q22 Are the following statements regarding bone marrow true or false?

(a) It is normal to see red bone marrow in the adult clavicle.
(b) MRI tends to underestimate the extent of red marrow activity.
(c) T2-weighted imaging is more sensitive than T1-weighted imaging for assessing bone marrow distribution.
(d) Regional migratory osteoporosis causes bone marrow fibrosis.
(e) Osteopetrosis results in reduction in both T1- and T2-weighted signal on MRI.

Q23 The following associations are correct. True or false?

(a) Medial meniscus – meniscocapsular separation.
(b) Lateral meniscus – discoid configuration more common.
(c) Patellar tendonitis – mid-portion of patellar tendon.
(d) Patella alta – achondroplasia.
(e) Iliotibial tract friction syndrome – medial aspect of the knee.

Q24 Are the following statements true or false?

(a) The anterior talofibular ligament inserts into the neck of the talus.

(b) The short plantar ligament extends from the calcaneum to the base of the metatarsals.
(c) The short saphenous vein passes anterior to the lateral malleolus.
(d) The peroneal artery divides into medial and lateral plantar branches.
(e) The dorsalis pedis artery passes between the first and second metatarsals to join the plantar arch.

Q25 Are the following statements regarding soft-tissue calcification true or false?

(a) Milk-alkali syndrome causes nephrocalcinosis.
(b) Dermatomyositis causes calcification along nerve sheaths.
(c) Parosteal lipoma is a recognised cause.
(d) Leprosy causes sheet-like calcification in the muscles.
(e) Alkaptonuria causes intervertebral disc calcification.

Q26 Are the following statements regarding the shoulder joint true or false?

(a) The glenohumeral ligaments are separate from the joint capsule.
(b) ALPSA implies avulsion of the inferior labrum.
(c) The Buford complex is associated with a thickened inferior glenohumeral ligament.
(d) Posterior glenohumeral instability is usually multi-directional.
(e) Medial subluxation of the biceps tendon is generally an isolated occurrence.

Q27 Are the following statements regarding the use of ultrasound in musculoskeletal radiology true or false?

(a) Tendon echogenicity is best assessed with the transducer perpendicular to the tendon.
(b) Pathology is generally echogenic.
(c) Articular cartilage is generally echo poor.

(d) The commonest cause of anterior elbow pain is rupture of the long head of biceps.

(e) A cross-sectional area of 15 mm^2 of the median nerve is normal.

Q28 The following anatomical variants are paired to their typical sites. True or false?

(a) Supracondylar process – humerus.
(b) Foramen – olecranon fossa.
(c) Accessory soleus muscle – thigh.
(d) Arcuate foramen – scaphoid bone.
(e) Ankle arthrogram – filling of the flexor hallucis longus tendon sheath.

Q29 The classification systems and pathologies given below are associated. True or false?

(a) Weber – knee fractures.
(b) Boyd–Griffin – pelvic fractures.
(c) Frykman – distal radial fractures.
(d) Ficat – avascular necrosis.
(e) D'Alonzo – odontoid peg fractures.

Q30 The following centring points are correct for each location. True or false?

(a) Lateral view of the foot – lateral cuneiform bone.
(b) Dorso-pedal view of the toes – head of third metatarsal.
(c) AP view of the pelvis – symphysis pubis.
(d) Lateral view of the lumbar spine – 10 cm anterior to the spinous process of the third lumbar vertebra.
(e) AP view of the shoulder – acromion process.

Q31 Are the following statements true or false? Pseudoarthrosis of the tibia and fibula:

(a) is associated with fibrous dysplasia.
(b) is associated with juvenile osteoporosis.
(c) is most commonly due to neurofibromatosis.
(d) typically arises at the junction of the mid and upper third.
(e) is easily treated.

Q32 The following radiological procedures and complications are associated. True or false?

(a) Arthrography – air embolism.
(b) Cervical spine discography – tonic/clonic seizure syndrome.
(c) Percutaneous vertebral biopsy – haemorrhage.
(d) Chemonucleolysis – cauda equina syndrome.
(e) Arthrography – synovial irritation.

Q33 The following can cause diffuse osteosclerosis. True or false?

(a) Mastocytosis.
(b) Multiple myeloma.
(c) Is a normal variant in neonates.
(d) Osteopoikilosis.
(e) Wilson's disease.

Q34 Are the following statements regarding multiple epiphyseal dysplasia true or false?

(a) It is inherited as autosomal dominant.
(b) It may result in increased height.
(c) It may be causative in early degenerative change.
(d) Multicentric ossification centres are a feature.
(e) The axial skeleton is generally involved.

(Q35) Nail–patella syndrome has the following features. True or false?

(a) Iliac horns.
(b) Dislocated radial head.
(c) Hypoplastic patellae.
(d) Thirteen ribs.
(e) Large parietal foramina of the skull.

(Q36) The following are causes of secondary hypertrophic pulmonary osteoarthropathy. True or false?

(a) Hodgkin's disease.
(b) Biliary atresia.
(c) Pachydermoperiostosis.
(d) Nasopharyngeal polyposis.
(e) Infected aortic grafts.

(Q37) Are the following statements regarding multicentric reticulohistiocytosis true or false?

(a) It is typified by osteopenia.
(b) It is associated with skin nodularity.
(c) It is due to infiltration by histiocytes.
(d) It is generally symmetrical.
(e) The metacarpophalangeal joints are generally the first involved.

(Q38) The following organisms/infectious diseases are correctly linked with their sequelae. True or false?

(a) Human immunodeficiency virus (HIV) – mycobacterium osteomyelitis.
(b) Actinomycosis – mandibular destruction.
(c) Brucellosis – intervertebral gas.
(d) Bone mycetoma – sclerosis.
(e) Viral infection – epiphyseal lucencies.

The following entities are normal findings/variants of the lower limb. True or false?

(a) Os acetabuli.
(b) Linea aspera.
(c) Peritendonitis calcarea.
(d) Os secundum.
(e) Fovea capitis.

 Are the following statements regarding the foot true or false?

(a) Os supratalare is found behind the talus.
(b) The calcaneus is most frequently fractured.
(c) Fractures of the anterior process of the calcaneum are typically avulsion injuries.
(d) Talar dislocations always occur with a fracture.
(e) Chopart's joint is found at the tarsometatarsal junction.

Answers

 (a) False.
(b) True.
(c) True.
(d) False.
(e) True.

A Hill–Sachs lesion is a fracture of the posterolateral aspect of the humeral head, resulting in a 'hatchet-like' defect and is best seen on internal rotation. There are three morphological types of acromion, namely type 1 (flat), type 2 (smoothly curved) and type 3 (hooked). The 40-degree posterior oblique view (Grashey view) reveals the normal space at the glenohumeral joint, which if obliterated raises the possibility of a posterior dislocation. A 15-degree cephalad tilt allows better assessment of the acromioclavicular joint. The lateral transthoracic, trans-scapular and axillary views all allow assessment of glenohumeral dislocation.

(a) True.
(b) True.
(c) False.
(d) True.
(e) False.

Erlenmeyer's flask deformity (bone distally expanded and thus shaped like a conical flask) usually affects the femur. It is almost always due to processes that expand the bone marrow. Other causes include Gaucher's and Niemann–Pick disease, anaemia, achondroplasia and Ollier's disease.

 (a) True.
(b) True.
(c) False.
(d) True.
(e) False.

Other benign musculoskeletal conditions with malignant potential are Paget's disease and chronic sinus tracts of osteomyelitis. The incidence of malignant change in the peripheral nerves of patients with neurofibromatosis is 3–16%. Secondary malignancy may also occur in patients with benign tumours such as enchondroma, osteochondroma and fibrous dysplasia.

 (a) False.
(b) True.
(c) False.
(d) False.
(e) False.

Tumoural calcinosis is an idiopathic disorder of periarticular calcium deposition. The deposits are painless and are commoner in children and adolescents. Causes of posterior vertebral scalloping may be subdivided as follows: increased intraspinal pressure (communicating hydrocephalus, intradural neoplasm); dural ectasia (Marfan's syndrome); congenital disorders (achondroplasia) and bone resorption (acromegaly).

Chondromyxoid fibroma is typically an expansile lytic lesion. Periosteal desmoid tumours are benign 'no-touch' lesions involving fibrous proliferation of the periosteum. They typically occur on the posteromedial aspect of the medial femoral condyle in patients between 12 and 20 years of age. Most disappear by the age of 20 years. Telangiectatic osteosarcoma is one of the more aggressive subtypes of osteosarcoma.

 A5 (a) False.
       (b) False.
       (c) True.
       (d) False.
       (e) False.

There are four fat planes adjacent to the hip joint in the medial space overlying the obturator internus and iliopsoas, and in the lateral spaces between gluteus minimus and medius, rectus femoris and tensor fasciae latae respectively. Displacement of the fat planes is a poor indicator of the presence or absence of joint swelling. Judet views are internal and external oblique views of the pelvis, which allow better assessment of the posterior acetabular rim. The inlet view is a 40–50-degree projection angled caudally and is good for evaluating sacral fractures. The mortality in pelvic fractures is between 9% and 19%. The Y vascular groove in the iliac bone is a normal variant, is marginated by sclerotic bone and is frequently bilateral.

 A6 (a) True.
       (b) False.
       (c) False.
       (d) False.
       (e) False.

At the wrist, the coronal axis is angled to allow adequate visualisation of the triangular fibrocartilage complex and intrinsic ligaments. STIR images are highly sensitive for bone bruising accompanying occult fractures. Sagittal images of the knee are obtained at an angle of 10 degrees anteromedially to the plane described. Sagittal oblique images are required for imaging the shoulder. Signal-to-noise ratio is reduced by 3-dimensional volume acquisition.

(a) False.
(b) False.
(c) True.
(d) False.
(e) False.

MFH is most commonly found in soft tissue and is often lytic on plain film. It is a rare diagnosis in the paediatric population and is usually photopenic on bone scan.

 (a) True.
(b) False.
(c) True.
(d) False.
(e) True.

Cortical desmoids are typically found on the posterior aspect of the medial femoral condyle. Chondroblastomas are usually benign and occur between 10 and 25 years of age. Osteofibrous dysplasia usually occurs in the tibia.

 (a) False.
(b) False.
(c) True.
(d) True.
(e) False.

One-third of Hodgkin's disease deposits are solitary. The vertebral end plate is often preserved. Lymphoblastic NHL spreads to bone as an early feature.

 (a) True.
(b) True.
(c) True.
(d) False.
(e) True.

Nowadays, dietary deficiency is an unusual cause of osteomalacia. Malabsorption and renal failure are commoner causes.

(A11) (a) False.
    (b) True.
    (c) True.
    (d) False.
    (e) True.

Inflammation of the enthesis (the osseous insertion of a tendon or ligament) results in bone proliferation and calcification at the insertion sites. It may also occur with diffuse idiopathic skeletal hyperostosis (DISH), ankylosing spondylitis and psoriatic arthropathy.

(A12) (a) True.
    (b) False.
    (c) False.
    (d) True.
    (e) False.

Hypervitaminosis A is usually seen in infants and causes pruritus, dry lips and skin, and hair loss. Hydrocephalus leads to cranial suture separation. Epiphyseal thinning and premature closure are seen as well as calcification within tendons and ligaments. Symmetrical periosteal new bone formation along the long bones is typical of hypervitaminosis A.

(A13) (a) True.
    (b) True.
    (c) True.
    (d) True.
    (e) True.

Abnormal joint mechanics post fracture predispose to osteoarthritis. Sudeck's atrophy (or reflex sympathetic dystrophy) may be idiopathic, or due to relatively trivial trauma, as well as myocardial infarction. Lead arthropathy is a rare complication of gunshot injuries. The lead fragments may become incorporated into the synovium, resulting in a degenerative arthritis, typically in unlucky grouse-beaters. Myositis ossificans is usually due to direct or repeated occupational trauma (e.g. fencers, riders).

(a) True.
(b) False.
(c) False.
(d) True.
(e) False.

Typical sites and causes of stress fractures include:

- Obturator ring – stooping/bowling/gymnastics.
- Lower cervical spine – clay shovelling.
- Sesamoids of metatarsals – prolonged standing.
- Hamate – golf/tennis/baseball.
- Pars interarticularis – ballet/ heavy lifting/scrubbing floors.
- Coracoid process of the scapula – trap shooting.
- Distal shaft of the humerus – throwing a ball.
- Coronoid process of the ulna – pitching a ball.
- Patella – hurdling.
- Proximal and distal parts of tibia/fibula – jumping and long distance running.

 (a) False.
(b) True.
(c) True.
(d) False.
(e) True.

Exuberant callus formation occurs in many conditions, especially where there is ineffective bone healing (steroids, Cushing's syndrome, multiple myeloma) or repeated trauma due to loss of sensation (congenital pain insensitivity, neuropathy).

 (a) True.
(b) True.
(c) False.
(d) False.
(e) True.

Although chondromyxoid fibroma is typically associated with a sclerotic reaction it does not demonstrate a periosteal reaction unless there is a fracture through it. Osseous MFH demonstrates a lamellated periosteal reaction although the lesion itself is lytic.

(a) False.
(b) True.
(c) False.
(d) False.
(e) True.

A Jefferson's fracture is a comminuted fracture of the C1 neural ring, involving both the anterior and posterior arches. The fracture is stable when the transverse ligament is intact and the total offset of the two sides is less than 7 mm. It is unstable when the offset is more than 7 mm, often with increased atlantoaxial distance on the lateral view. Fifty-five per cent of C2 injuries are odontoid peg fractures, and 25% are hangman fractures (bilateral fractures of the neural arch). The ring of C2 is only disrupted in type III dens fractures. A teardrop fracture is a comminuted fracture of the vertebral body with a characteristic triangular fragment from the anterior inferior portion. In 50% of cases, a vertical sagittal split may be seen on the anteroposterior (AP) view on plain film.

 (a) False.
(b) False.
(c) True.
(d) False.
(e) False.

Bennett's (and Rolando's) fractures are intra-articular. Fractures of the sesamoid bone of the thumb are usually horizontal. The commonest metacarpal base fractures are at the fourth and fifth fingers. Dorsal interphalangeal dislocation is much more common than volar.

 (a) False.
(b) True.
(c) True.
(d) True.
(e) False.

The avulsion fracture associated with an ACL tear arises from the anterior tibial eminence. The ACL normally limits anterior tibial translation and hyperextension. Bone bruising is typically in the posterolateral tibial plateau.

 (a) True.
    (b) True.
    (c) True.
    (d) True.
    (e) False.

Elastofibroma is a benign tumour secondary to mechanical friction; it is bilateral in 25%. The muscle most commonly affected by focal herniation through the fascial defect is the tibialis anterior. This often requires surgical repair. Aggressive extra-abdominal fibromatosis is a benign aggressively growing soft-tissue neoplasm. Seventy per cent grow in the extremities and 75% recur within two years of surgery. MRI is poor at completely distinguishing lipomatous tumours, however, the sarcomatous variety does enhance after intravenous contrast.

 (a) True.
    (b) True.
    (c) False.
    (d) False.
    (e) True.

The posterior tibial nerve may be entrapped at the ankle joint and the anterior tibial nerve at the proximal fibula. The suprascapular nerve typically may be compromised at the suprascapular notch, which is located on the superior aspect of the scapula, below the transverse ligament.

 (a) True.
    (b) True.
    (c) False.
    (d) False.
    (e) True.

Normal sites for red bone marrow in the adult include the bones of the skull, vertebral column, thoracic cage, pelvic girdle, and the head of the humerus and femur. T1-weighted imaging is superior to

T2-weighted for bone marrow imaging. Regional migratory osteo-porosis causes bone marrow oedema.

 (a)   True.
(b)   True.
(c)   False.
(d)   False.
(e)   False.

The medial meniscus is attached to the deep fibres of the medial collateral ligament and may become detached from the latter in traumatic injury; the lateral meniscus is not attached to the lateral collateral ligament. Discoid configuration is much more common in the lateral meniscus and more liable to tear. Patellar tendonitis usually occurs at the inferior or superior aspect of the tendon (jumper's knee). Patella baja (low lying) is associated with achondroplasia. The iliotibial tract is situated on the lateral aspect of the knee.

 (a)   True.
(b)   False.
(c)   False.
(d)   False.
(e)   True.

The anterior, posterior and calcaneofibular ligaments stabilise the lateral part of the ankle. The short plantar ligament extends from the calcaneum to the base of the cuboid, the long plantar ligament extends to the base of the metatarsals. The short saphenous vein passes posterior to the lateral malleolus. The posterior tibial artery divides into medial and lateral plantar branches.

 (a)   True.
(b)   False.
(c)   True.
(d)   False.
(e)   True.

Dermatomyositis causes sheet-like calcification in the muscles, and leprosy causes calcification along the nerve sheaths. Alkaptonuria also causes calcification in the pinna of the ear and periarticular soft tissues.

 (a) False.
(b) False.
(c) False.
(d) True.
(e) False.

The glenohumeral ligaments fuse with the anterior surface of the shoulder capsule. The ALPSA lesion is an avulsion of the anterior labroligamentous periosteal sleeve. The Buford complex is a normal variant in which a cord-like middle glenohumeral ligament is found with absence of the anterosuperior portion of the glenoid labrum. Subluxation of the biceps tendon is unusual without a rotator cuff tear.

 (a) False.
(b) False.
(c) True.
(d) True.
(e) False.

If the transducer is not parallel to the tendon, beam anisotropy may occur with a spurious appearance of increased echogenicity. Pathology is generally echo poor. A cross-sectional area of 15 mm² in the proximal part of the carpal tunnel is pathological, implying carpal tunnel syndrome.

 (a) True.
(b) True.
(c) False.
(d) False.
(e) True.

The accessory soleus muscle is found in the calf. The arcuate foramen is sited in the posterior arch of the C1 vertebra. Filling of the flexor hallucis and digitorum tendon sheath spaces as well as the posterior subtalar joint space occurs normally in 20% and 10% of ankle arthrograms, respectively.

(a) False.
(b) False.
(c) True.
(d) True.
(e) True.

Weber's classification grades ankle fractures according to the level of fibular fracture and presence or absence of associated medial malleolar fracture. The Boyd–Griffin classification grades inter-trochanteric fractures according to the degree of comminution and involvement of the subtrochanteric region. Frykman's classification grades distal radial fractures according to location of fracture line and presence of ulnar fracture.

 (a) False.
(b) True.
(c) False.
(d) True.
(e) False.

Centring points:

- Lateral view of the foot – cuboid bone.
- The AP view of the pelvis is centred 5 cm above the midline of the symphysis pubis.
- AP view of the shoulder – coracoid process.

 (a) True.
(b) True.
(c) True.
(d) False.
(e) False.

Pseudoarthrosis typically occurs in the mid- and lower-third of the tibia. It is difficult to treat. Pseudoarthrosis may also occur in the clavicle and forearm.

 (a) True.
(b) True.
(c) True.

(d) True.

(e) True.

The reported complications of the following procedures include:

- Arthrography – infection, synovial irritation, allergic reactions, syncope and air embolism.
- Discography – misplacement of the needle and infection.
- Percutaneous vertebral biopsy – pneumothorax, nerve root damage, cord damage and haemorrhage.
- Chemonucleolysis – allergic reactions, disc infection, neurological complications including raised intracranial pressure, paraplegia, and cauda equina syndrome.

 (a) True.

(b) True.

(c) True.

(d) False.

(e) False.

Diffuse osteosclerosis is found in neonates, particularly if premature. Osteopoikilosis generally causes punctuate areas of increased sclerosis. Wilson's disease generally results in diffuse osteopenia.

 (a) True.

(b) False.

(c) True.

(d) True.

(e) False.

Short stature is a feature of multiple epiphyseal dysplasia, with short stubby fingers found as an association. The ossification centres fuse prematurely. The adjacent metaphyses are often broadened. The axial skeleton is generally normal, however, Schmorl's nodes or a Scheurmann-like appearance may be present.

 (a) True.

(b) False.

(c) True.

(d) False.

(e) True.

Nail–patella syndrome is transmitted as autosomal dominant. Its associations include: hypoplastic radial head, 11 pairs of ribs, Madelung's deformity of the wrist, muscular hypoplasia, disorders of the iris, renal abnormalities and hypertension.

 (a) True.
(b) True.
(c) False.
(d) False.
(e) True.

Pachydermoperiostosis is the primary form (of hypertrophic osteo-arthropathy) and has autosomal dominant transmission, accounting for 2–3% of cases. It typically occurs in black men, resulting in finger clubbing, generalised pachydermia and excessive sweating. Nasopharyngeal carcinoma may result in this radiological finding, as well as gastrointestinal polyposis.

 (a) False.
(b) True.
(c) True.
(d) True.
(e) False.

Multicentric reticulohistiocytosis results in widespread, symmetrical and progressive arthropathy, beginning in the wrists and interphalangeal joints, and spreading to the metacarpophalangeal joints. Erosions tend to be large and punched out. Arthritis mutilans may result.

 (a) True.
(b) True.
(c) True.
(d) False.
(e) True.

The mandible is the bone most commonly affected by actinomycosis. Brucellosis may occur as a synovitis, spondylitis (producing gas) or arthritis. Mycetoma is due to direct infection by fungi, resulting in chronic osteomyelitis and lytic expanded areas.

(a) True.
        (b) True.
        (c) True.
        (d) False.
        (e) True.

Os acetabuli is an accessory ossification centre at the superolateral aspect of the acetabulum. The linea aspera is a line found in the posterior distal third of the femur. Peritendonitis calcarea is an amorphous area of calcification overlying the greater trochanter. Os secundum is an accessory bone in the hand. The fovea capitis is found in the femoral head.

 (a) False.
        (b) True.
        (c) True.
        (d) False.
        (e) False.

Os supratalare is found anterosuperior to the talus. Talar dislocations may occur without a fracture. Chopart's joint is at the talonavicular and calcaneocuboid levels.

Section 4

Gastrointestinal and hepatobiliary

Q1 The following conditions are associated with stomach polyps. True or false?

(a) Peutz–Jegher's syndrome.
(b) Cowden's disease.
(c) Turcot's syndrome.
(d) Chronic gastritis.
(e) Familial polyposis coli.

Q2 The differential diagnosis of thickened oesophageal folds includes the following conditions. True or false?

(a) Lymphoma.
(b) Oesophageal papillomatosis.
(c) Varicoid carcinoma.
(d) Oesophagitis.
(e) Leukoplakia.

Q3 Are the following statements true or false?

(a) Embryologically, the ventral pancreatic bud forms the head and uncinate pancreas.
(b) The inferior rectal vein drains into the inferior mesenteric vein.
(c) The cystic duct normally lies posterior to the common hepatic duct.

69

(d) The bare area of the liver is bounded by the triangular ligaments.

(e) The ureter lies medial to the duct for the vas deferens on the posterior aspect of the bladder.

Q4 The following are relative and absolute contraindications to percutaneous gastrostomy. True or false?

(a) Anoxic brain injury.
(b) Previous gastric surgery.
(c) Portal hypertension with varices.
(d) Severe pulmonary disease.
(e) Interposed bowel.

Q5 Are the following statements regarding cholangiocarcinomas true or false?

(a) Choledochal cysts are a risk factor for their development.
(b) They are generally squamous carcinomas.
(c) They are commoner among men.
(d) Less than 30% are located at the liver hilum.
(e) Complications are more common via the endoscopic than the transhepatic route of biliary drainage.

Q6 Are the following statements regarding the imaging features of hepatocellular carcinoma (HCC) true or false?

(a) Capsular invasion occurs in 10%.
(b) The tumour is calcified in 50%.
(c) The presence of portal venous tumour is non-specific in the diagnosis.
(d) Brain metastases are found in association with lung metastases.
(e) The tumour capsule is hypoechoic on ultrasound.

The following are features of endometrial carcinoma on ultrasound. True or false?

(a) Endometrial thickness greater than 10 mm.
(b) The thickened endometrium is hyperechoic.
(c) The arterial flow demonstrates a high resistive index.
(d) Myometrial invasion may be suggested by disruption of the subendometrial hypoechoic layer.
(e) In young women, the endometrial thickness should not exceed 8 mm.

 The following lesions may present as cystic lesions of the spleen. True or false?

(a) Gaucher's disease.
(b) Haematoma.
(c) Haemangioma.
(d) Epidermoid cyst.
(e) Infarct.

 Are the following statements true or false?

(a) Primary lipomas of the liver are associated with tuberous sclerosis.
(b) The von Meyenburg complex is due to failure of involution of embryonic hepatocytes.
(c) Cystic fibrosis is associated with hyperplasia of the gallbladder.
(d) Dilatation of the pancreatic duct is a feature of acute pancreatic transplant rejection.
(e) The normal deployed diameter of a transjugular intrahepatic portosystemic shunt (TIPS) stent is 8–10 mm.

 The following are causes of hepatic arterio-portal shunting. True or false?

(a) Hepatocellular carcinoma.
(b) Congenital.

(c)   Trauma.
(d)   Gaucher's disease.
(e)   Hepatic adenoma.

(Q11)   Are the following statements regarding liver transplantation true or false?

(a)   Primary hepatocellular carcinoma is an indication for liver transplantation.
(b)   Hepatic arterial thrombosis is the commonest vascular complication post transplantation.
(c)   Portal vein occlusion occurs commonly.
(d)   Non-anastomotic biliary strictures have a good prognosis.
(e)   Non-Hodgkin's lymphoma may occur as a complication.

(Q12)   Are the following statements regarding pancreatic carcinoma true or false?

(a)   Peripancreatic lymphadenopathy precludes resectability.
(b)   Superior mesenteric involvement implies unresectability.
(c)   Pancreatic atrophy is an early sign.
(d)   The pancreas is best imaged at 40 seconds post intravenous contrast.
(e)   Tumours of over 3 cm are generally operable.

(Q13)   The following mesenteric neoplasms are benign. True or false?

(a)   Mesenteric lipodystrophy.
(b)   Lipoma.
(c)   Mesenteric cyst.
(d)   Neurofibroma.
(e)   Peritoneal mesothelioma.

Q14 The following conditions are abdominal manifestations of acquired immune deficiency syndrome (AIDS). True or false?

(a) Peliosis hepatis.
(b) Cholangiopathy.
(c) Enteropathy.
(d) Cholangiocarcinoma.
(e) CMV (cytomegalovirus) colitis.

Q15 The following conditions are found in patients with chronic renal failure. True or false?

(a) Spontaneous colonic perforation.
(b) Gastritis.
(c) Oesophageal varices.
(d) Pseudomembranous colitis.
(e) Pancreatitis.

Q16 The following conditions are associated with an increased incidence of malignancy. True or false?

(a) Porcelain gallbladder.
(b) Gallbladder polyp >1 cm.
(c) Pancreatic divisum.
(d) Chronic pancreatitis.
(e) Glycogen storage disease.

Q17 Are the following statements regarding biliary cystadenoma true or false?

(a) It has a peak incidence in the second decade.
(b) It is managed conservatively by serial imaging.
(c) It is a multiloculated cystic tumour.
(d) It is hypervascular on angiography.
(e) It most commonly arises from the extrahepatic biliary tree.

Q18 Are the following statements regarding Budd–Chiari syndrome true or false?

(a) It is idiopathic in 30% of cases.
(b) It is always due to thrombosis.
(c) Caudate hypertrophy is present in 40% of cases.
(d) The portal vein diameter typically increases.
(e) Paroxysmal nocturnal haemoglobinuria is a risk factor.

Q19 Simultaneous involvement of the gastric antrum and bulb may occur in the following conditions. True or false?

(a) Crohn's disease.
(b) Eosinophilic gastroenteritis.
(c) Varices.
(d) Brunner's gland hyperplasia.
(e) Tuberculosis.

Q20 Are the following statements regarding contrast agents true or false?

(a) Levovist, a microbubble contrast agent, improves specificity of identification of hepatic metastases.
(b) There is loss of signal on T2-weighted magnetic resonance imaging (MRI) of focal nodular hyperplasia, after administration of SPIO (super paramagnetic iron oxide particles).
(c) Delayed-enhanced CT is irrelevant in the diagnosis of adrenal adenomas.
(d) Gadolinium-enhanced magnetic resonance angiography (MRA) is useful in pre-renal transplant assessment.
(e) Bubble noise is a recognised artefact of microbubble use.

Q21 The following anatomical arrangements are most commonly found. True or false?

(a) The right hepatic artery is posterior to the common hepatic duct.

(b)   The right hepatic artery is posterior to the portal vein.
(c)   The cystic artery crosses anterior to the common hepatic duct.
(d)   The tip of the appendix is closely related to the terminal ileum.
(e)   The oesophageal hiatus lies at the level of the T12 vertebra.

(Q22)   The following are recognised normal variants. True or false?

(a)   Separate insertion of the right hepatic vein into the inferior vena cava.
(b)   A left hepatic artery arising from the superior mesenteric artery.
(c)   Intrahepatic gallbladder.
(d)   Separate opening of the common bile duct and pancreatic duct.
(e)   The right gastric artery supplying the ascending colon.

(Q23)   Are the following statements regarding the adrenal glands true or false?

(a)   They are enclosed in perirenal fascia.
(b)   The right adrenal has a larger medial limb.
(c)   The right gland is typically Y shaped.
(d)   They are one-third the size of the kidney at birth.
(e)   Cortical bodies are recognised normal aberrant rests of adrenal tissue.

(Q24)   Are the following statements regarding diagnostic ultrasound true or false?

(a)   It relies on the different acoustic impedance of tissues to produce an image.
(b)   Time gain compensation can be used to even out an ultrasound appearance.
(c)   A standard transducer frequency for abdominal scanning is 10 MHz.

(d) Acoustic enhancement is worsened by time gain compensation.
(e) Local heating is a recognised side effect.

Q25 Are the following statements regarding MRI of the abdomen and pelvis true or false?

(a) Out of phase T1-weighted imaging is useful in the diagnosis of fatty liver.
(b) HASTE is typically a T1-weighted sequence.
(c) Fat suppression is superior without gadolinium enhancement for the detection of pathology.
(d) Motion artefact is more pronounced in the phase-encoding direction.
(e) Reduction of the field of view improves spatial resolution.

Q26 Are the following statements regarding CT of the gastrointestinal and genitourinary tracts true or false?

(a) It is excellent at defining the T stage of oesophageal tumours.
(b) The oesophageal wall measures 3 mm.
(c) It can be difficult to detect peritoneal and omental deposits.
(d) Local staging of rectal cancer is better with introduction of rectal air.
(e) If the fat plane is preserved around an adrenal tumour, this is a poor indicator of the absence of local invasion.

Q27 The following are recognised complications of barium enema as a procedure. True or false?

(a) Perforation.
(b) Portal vein embolisation.
(c) Diarrhoea.
(d) Vaginal rupture.
(e) Septicaemia.

The differential diagnosis of hepatic calcification includes the following. True or false?

(a) Hydatid disease.
(b) Sarcoidosis.
(c) Portal vein thrombosis.
(d) Ovarian metastases.
(e) Chronic granulomatous disease of childhood.

 Are the following statements regarding colitis true or false?

(a) Acute cases may demonstrate a narrowed prerectal space.
(b) Fibrofatty proliferation of the pericolic fat is recognised.
(c) Aphthoid ulceration is found in ulcerative colitis.
(d) Schistosomiasis is a cause in the large bowel.
(e) It most commonly occurs in the ileocaecal region in Behçet's syndrome.

 Are the following statements regarding abdominal lymphoma true or false?

(a) Mesenteric nodes are common in Hodgkin's disease.
(b) Splenic nodal involvement is commonly associated with splenic infiltration.
(c) Contiguous spread is a feature of Hodgkin's disease.
(d) T cell neoplasms are more common histologically.
(e) Radiotherapy is used for stage 1 disease.

 Are the following statements regarding splenic pathology true or false?

(a) Splenic angiosarcoma is the commonest non-lymphoid primary malignant tumour.
(b) Breast malignancy is a recognised cause of splenic deposits.
(c) Fungal infection of the spleen is typically miliary.
(d) Haemosiderosis of the spleen results in increased T2-weighted signal on MRI.

(e) Acute splenic sequestration on CT has the typical appearance of splenomegaly and peripheral low attenuation regions in keeping with infarction.

(Q32) Abdominal lymphadenopathy with a low density centre may occur with the following. True or false?

(a) *Mycobacterium avium-intracellulare.*
(b) Whipple's disease.
(c) Crohn's disease.
(d) Neurofibromatosis I.
(e) Lymphangioleiomyomatosis.

(Q33) Are the following statements regarding cholangitis true or false?

(a) Ampullary carcinoma is a risk factor.
(b) It is suppurative in 90%.
(c) It may result in transient periportal hyperaemia on arterial phase CT imaging.
(d) Secondary sclerosing cholangitis is a complication.
(e) It may be caused by chemotherapy.

(Q34) Are the following statements true or false? On MRI:

(a) T2-weighted images are useful in the diagnosis of intestinal atresia.
(b) Small bowel leiomyomas typically do not enhance with gadolinium.
(c) GIST gastric tumours typically have hypervascular liver metastases.
(d) Desmoplastic reaction secondary to carcinoid results in reduced T1- and T2-weighted signals.
(e) The severity of Crohn's disease may be assessed.

(Q35) Are the following statements true or false?

(a) An accessory lobe of the parotid occurs in 20%.
(b) The submandibular space contains the facial artery.

(c) Perineural invasion is atypical for adenoid cystic carcinoma.
(d) Parotid involvement is associated with a worse prognosis in HIV-positive children.
(e) Warthin's tumour typically occurs in the parotid gland.

Q36 Adrenal calcification may be due to the following causes. True or false?

(a) Wolman's disease.
(b) Adrenocortical carcinoma.
(c) Haemorrhage.
(d) Rhabdomyosarcoma.
(e) Phaeochromocytoma.

Q37 Are the following statements regarding CT colonography true or false?

(a) All mobile lesions are faecal material.
(b) Polyps are generally of homogeneous attenuation.
(c) It is readily able to diagnose lesions 4–6 mm in size.
(d) Flat adenomas are easily missed.
(e) The ideal section is 4 mm thick.

Q38 Are the following statements regarding oesophageal pathology true or false?

(a) Peptic strictures are generally longer than 4 mm.
(b) Strictures post-nasogastic intubation only occur after a long period.
(c) Barrett's oesophagus may cause the stricture in the mid-portion.
(d) Epidermolysis bullosa typically affects the lower oesophagus.
(e) Post-radiotherapy strictures appear within the first year after treatment.

The following lesions may occur in the appendix. True or false?

(a) Kaposi's sarcoma.
(b) Adenoma.
(c) Lymphoma.
(d) Signet cell tumour.
(e) Malignant fibrous histiocytoma.

 Emphysema may occur in the following organs. True or false?

(a) Bladder.
(b) Pancreas.
(c) Gallbladder.
(d) Adrenal glands.
(e) Uterus.

Answers

 (a) True.
(b) True.
(c) False.
(d) True.
(e) True.

Peutz–Jegher's syndrome is an autosomal dominant inherited disease characterised by mucocutaneous pigmentation and gastrointestinal polyps. The polyps occur in the small bowel (90%), colon (30%), stomach (25%) and duodenum (15%). Those in the stomach and small bowel are usually hamartomas, whereas the colonic polyps are adenomatous with malignant potential. Cowden's disease is a rare autosomal dominant disease with endodermal, mesodermal and ectodermal abnormalities. Small sessile polyps are found throughout the gastrointestinal tract. Turcot's syndrome is an autosomal recessive colonic polyposis associated with tumours of the central nervous system, especially medulloblastoma and glioblastoma. Chronic gastritis is associated with the development of gastric polyps. Familial polyposis coli is associated with multiple adenomatous polyps and has an autosomal dominant inheritance.

 A2   (a) True.
       (b) False.
       (c) True.
       (d) True.
       (e) False.

Oesophageal papillomatosis and leukoplakia typically produce multiple nodules.

 A3   (a) True.
       (b) False.
       (c) True.
       (d) True.
       (e) False.

In embryological development, the ventral pancreas forms the head and the dorsal pancreas forms the body and tail. The inferior rectal vein drains into the common iliac veins. The cystic duct normally lies posterior to the common hepatic duct, although if its insertion is more inferior it tends to cross anteriorly – which is of importance to the surgeon when ligating the cystic duct. The ureter lies lateral to the vas deferens duct.

 A4   (a) False.
       (b) True.
       (c) True.
       (d) False.
       (e) True.

Previous gastric surgery may render a percutaneous approach difficult or impossible. The presence of varices considerably increases the risks of the procedure and may necessitate an endoscopic or combined approach. Interposed bowel should be actively excluded before gastric puncture.

 A5   (a) True.
       (b) False.
       (c) True.

(d) False.
(e) False.

Risk factors for development of cholangiocarcinoma include: primary sclerosing cholangitis, hepatolithiasis, ulcerative colitis, biliary parasites, specific oncogenes and congenital malformations such as choledochal cysts. Cholangiocarcinomas are generally adenocarcinomas and are more common in men. Two-thirds are located at the liver hilum. During treatment, complications occur more commonly via the transhepatic than the endoscopic route.

A6 (a) False.
     (b) False.
     (c) False.
     (d) True.
     (e) True.

Capsular invasion occurs in 40% of HCC. There is portal vein invasion in 60% at autopsy, which is an important clue in the diagnosis of HCC, as less than 8% of portal vein tumours are due to other malignancies. It calcifies in 2–12% of cases. Brain metastases are hypervascular and usually occur in conjunction with lung metastases, whereas metastases of the skull base or vault are rare, usually expansile and are associated with other skeletal deposits. Most HCC that are 1 cm in diameter are homogeneous and hypoechoic in echo texture, which is non-specific. As the tumour enlarges, it becomes more inhomogeneous.

A7 (a) True.
     (b) True.
     (c) False.
     (d) True.
     (e) False.

On ultrasound, endometrial carcinoma appears as hyperechoic and heterogeneous in echo texture with a thickness between 10 and 20 mm. The arterial flow demonstrates a low resistive index (<0.4) and an elevated peak systolic velocity. In young women, the endometrium may measure up to 15 mm depending on the phase of the menstrual cycle. In post-menopausal women, this measures up to 5 mm, however, if on additional tamoxifen or HRT, it may measure up to 8 mm.

 (a) False.
(b) True.
(c) False.
(d) True.
(e) True.

Gaucher's disease presents with multiple low attenuation nodules within the spleen. Mature haematomas become cystic and haemangiomas are solid.

 (a) True.
(b) False.
(c) False.
(d) True.
(e) True.

The von Meyenburg complex (multiple bile duct hamartomas) is due to failure of involution of embryonic bile ducts, resulting in the appearance of multiple small cysts up to 10 mm in size. Cystic fibrosis is associated with hypoplasia of the gallbladder.

 (a) True.
(b) True.
(c) True.
(d) False.
(e) False.

Hepatic arterio-portal shunting may be congenital. It may be seen in malignancy and after trauma (including liver biopsy).

 (a) True.
(b) True.
(c) False.
(d) False.
(e) True.

Portal vein occlusion occurs rarely (in 2% of cases). Non-anastomotic strictures carry a poor prognosis due to their association with hepatic arterial thrombosis in 50% of cases.

 A12
    (a) False.
    (b) True.
    (c) True.
    (d) True.
    (e) False.

The following signs imply unresectability: metastases; extensive lymphadenopathy beyond the peripancreatic chain; malignant ascites/effusion; peritoneal deposits; vascular encasement; occlusion or alteration in contour or calibre; and contiguity between tumour and major vessel >50%. The presence of smaller tumours may be implied by the identification of a change in the normal biconcave margin of the uncinate process, pancreatic and biliary duct dilatation and pancreatic atrophy. Tumours over 3 cm are generally not considered operable as the outcome has a direct correlation with tumour size.

 A13
    (a) True.
    (b) True.
    (c) True.
    (d) True.
    (e) False.

Mesenteric lipodystrophy is a rare disorder causing fibrofatty thickening and fibrosis of the small bowel mesentery. Although associated with gastric and colonic carcinoma, it is not itself malignant. Peritoneal mesothelioma is associated with asbestos exposure, is highly malignant and carries a very poor prognosis.

 A14
    (a) True.
    (b) True.
    (c) True.
    (d) False.
    (e) True.

Peliosis hepatis is a rare condition characterised by sinusoidal dilatation and multiple blood-filled cystic lesions of the liver. It is also associated with malignancy, tuberculosis, and chronic steroid use. It is thought to be due to infection by a bacterium, *Rochalimaea henselae*. AIDS cholangitis is an acalculous inflammation resulting from opportunistic infection with Cryptosporidium and cytomegalovirus (CMV). Enteropathy may be due to direct infection by the HIV virus.

 (a) True.
(b) True.
(c) False.
(d) True.
(e) True.

Spontaneous colonic perforation is thought to be due to increased ischaemia and diverticulosis. Gastritis is commoner because of altered gastrin and gastric acid levels. Pseudomembranous, ischaemic and non-specific uraemic colitis are all common. Pancreatitis is commoner because of hypercalcaemia and use of immunosuppressives and steroids.

 (a) True.
(b) True.
(c) False.
(d) True.
(e) True.

Porcelain gallbladder carries a 10–20% risk of developing carcinoma. Of patients with chronic pancreatitis 2–4% go on to develop carcinoma. Glycogen storage disease has an increased incidence of HCC and hepatic adenoma.

 (a) False.
(b) False.
(c) True.
(d) False.
(e) False.

The peak incidence of biliary cystadenoma occurs in the fifth decade, and it is generally surgically resected due to the risk of malignant transformation to cystadenocarcinoma. It is hypovascular on angiography and most commonly arises from the intrahepatic biliary tree.

 (a) False.
(b) False.
(c) False.
(d) True.
(e) True.

Budd–Chiari syndrome is idiopathic in 70% of cases. Non-thrombotic causes of obstruction include tumour ingrowth, membrane or web, constrictive pericarditis and right heart failure. Thrombotic causes include polycythaemia, thrombocytosis, oral contraceptive pill, pregnancy, and paroxysmal nocturnal haemoglobinuria. Caudate lobe hypertrophy is present in 80–90% of cases.

 (a) True.
(b) True.
(c) False.
(d) False.
(e) True.

Varices from portal hypertension may be seen at the oesophagogastric junction, lesser curve, duodenum (from the posterior superior pancreaticoduodenal vein). Eosinophilic gastroenteritis usually affects the gastric antrum but can also affect the bulb. Brunner's gland hyperplasia affects the antrum and proximal two-thirds of the duodenum.

 (a) True.
(b) True.
(c) False.
(d) True.
(e) True.

Levovist-enhanced ultrasound has been shown to improve sensitivity and specificity of the detection of hepatic metastases. Focal nodular hyperplasia typically demonstrates hypo- or iso-intensity on T2-weighted MRI after administration of SPIO (super paramagnetic iron oxide particles). Delayed Hounsfield unit measurements are used for differentiation of adrenal adenomas and carcinomas. Gadolinium-enhanced MRA is a useful non-invasive means of establishing vascular and renal anatomy before renal transplant. Bubble noise is a recognised artefact due to breakdown of microbubbles and larger bubbles during insonation.

 (A21)   (a)   True.
    (b)   True.
    (c)   False.
    (d)   False.
    (e)   False.

The cystic artery is normally posterior to the common hepatic duct and crosses anteriorly when a low insertion into the hepatic artery occurs. The tip of the appendix is situated close to the terminal ileum in only 1% of cases. The oesophageal hiatus is situated at the level of the T10 vertebra.

 (A22)   (a)   True.
    (b)   True.
    (c)   True.
    (d)   True.
    (e)   False.

Intrahepatic gallbladder is normal in the fetus up to two months in utero. The common hepatic duct and pancreatic duct may have a separate opening in 50% of cases.

 (A23)   (a)   True.
    (b)   True.
    (c)   False.
    (d)   True.
    (e)   True.

Both adrenal glands are enclosed within the perirenal fascia but are separated from the kidney by perirenal fat. Although both glands are usually described as inverted Y in shape, the left appear as an inverted V because of the shortening of one of the limbs.

(A24) (a) True.
       (b) True.
       (c) False.
       (d) True.
       (e) True.

The acoustic impedance of a tissue is related to its density; the greater the mismatch in acoustic impedance between two adjacent tissues the more reflective will be their boundary. Usual frequency for scanning abdominal viscera is 3.5–5 MHz. During scanning, tissue is heated through contact with the imaging transducer and by absorption of the ultrasound energy.

(A25) (a) True.
       (b) False.
       (c) False.
       (d) True.
       (e) True.

Out-of-phase imaging results from the slight difference in resonance frequencies of the protons. It causes black 'outlining' of tissues and decrease in signal from voxels containing both water and fat. At 1.5 T, the water and fat signals are in phase when time to echo (TE) is an even multiple, and out of phase when TE is an odd multiple of 2.3 ms. The HASTE (half Fourier acquisition single shot turbo spin echo) sequence is typically a T2-weighted sequence. Fat suppression in combination with gadolinium enhancement is superior to non-enhancement. Motion artefact occurs in the phase-encoding direction. As the field of view is reduced, the voxel size becomes smaller and the resolution higher, but the measured signal decreases.

(a) False.
   (b) True.
   (c) True.
   (d) True.
   (e) False.

CT is poor at defining the level of invasion of oesophageal tumours. Peritoneal and omental deposits are often understaged on CT. Insufflation of air into the rectum aids appreciation of the extent of wall thickening.

 (a) True.
   (b) True.
   (c) False.
   (d) True.
   (e) True.

Perforation is less common with barium enema than colonoscopy. Bacteraemia, endocarditis, septicaemia and portal vein embolisation have all been described.

 (a) True.
   (b) False.
   (c) True.
   (d) True.
   (e) True.

Hydatid disease typically causes crescentic or curvilinear calcification in the pericyst, and it is commoner in the right lobe. Portal vein thrombus may itself calcify or there may be calcification in the portal vein wall. Ovarian metastases may calcify (as well as colonic and osteosarcoma metastases).

 (a) False.
   (b) True.
   (c) False.
   (d) True.
   (e) True.

Acute ulcerative colitis expands the presacral space but this may become narrowed in chronic cases. Compared with ulcerative colitis, Crohn's disease is usually worse in the right colon with sparing of the sigmoid and rectum. Fistulas (in ano, or colonic parallel to the bowel lumen) and deep ulcers are commoner. In the gastrointestinal tract, schistosomiasis is associated with hepatic fibrosis and portal hypertension, varices, granulomatous colitis and colonic strictures. Behçet's syndrome can cause ulceration anywhere in the gastrointestinal tract.

(a) False.
(b) True.
(c) True.
(d) False.
(e) True.

Mesenteric nodes and non-contiguous spread are more typical of non-Hodgkin's lymphoma.

(a) True.
(b) True.
(c) True.
(d) False.
(e) True.

Splenic angiosarcoma is a very rare tumour with a poor prognosis. Iron deposits in spleen or liver cause low T2 signal. Splenic sequestration crisis is an early manifestation of sickle cell disease which presents occasionally. Post-mortems demonstrate a massively enlarged spleen with an accumulation of sickled erythrocytes trapped within the splenic sinusoids.

(a) True.
(b) True.
(c) False.
(d) False.
(e) False.

Abdominal lymphadenopathy with a low-density centre may also be seen with lymphoma and pyogenic infections.

(A33) (a) True.
(b) False.
(c) True.
(d) True.
(e) True.

Ampullary carcinoma or consequences of chemotherapy may alter bile flow and precipitate cholangitis. In most cases the cholangitis is non-suppurative and the patient is not septicaemic. The increased contrast enhancement is more marked in the extrahepatic portal vessels. Secondary sclerosing cholangitis is a complication of chronic cholangitis.

(A34) (a) True.
(b) False.
(c) True.
(d) True.
(e) True.

T2 coronal images may be particularly helpful in appreciating the atretic bowel segment. Small bowel leiomyomas are hypervascular and enhance with contrast. The dense fibrosis within desmoplasia secondary to carcinoid results in reduced signal on T1- and T2-weighted images.

(A35) (a) True.
(b) False.
(c) False.
(d) False.
(e) True.

The submandibular space contains the lingual artery. Adenoid cystic carcinoma of the parotid tends to spread along the facial nerve. Parotitis is commonly seen in HIV-positive children. Warthin's tumour is relatively common and benign.

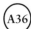(A36) (a) True.
(b) True.
(c) True.

(d) False.
(e) True.

Wolman's disease is a rare autosomal inherited lipidosis, which results in enlarged adrenals with bilateral punctuate calcification (highly diagnostic appearance). Adrenocortical carcinoma calcifies only occasionally, but if it does this is suggestive of malignancy. Phaeochromocytoma calcifies in 10% of cases.

 (a) False.
(b) True.
(c) False.
(d) True.
(e) False.

Polyps may also be mobile, so mobility on turning the patient can be falsely reassuring. At the time of writing, CT colonography is readily able to diagnose lesions greater than 10 mm in size; below this the sensitivity drops significantly. The ideal section thickness is 1.25 mm. Flat adenomas may be more easily recognisable with virtual colonoscopy.

 (a) True.
(b) False.
(c) True.
(d) False.
(e) True.

Strictures are considered to be over 10 mm in length. Benign peptic strictures are usually longer than malignant ones. Strictures post-nasogastric intubation may occur after three days. Epidermolysis bullosa typically affects the upper oesophagus. Post-radiotherapy strictures appear 4–8 months after treatment.

 (a) True.
(b) True.
(c) True.
(d) False.
(e) False.

Kaposi's sarcoma occurs in the skin, lymph nodes, liver, lungs and anywhere in the gastrointestinal tract. Signet cell tumour is a mucinous variant of adenocarcinoma usually arising in the colon or stomach. Malignant fibrous histiocytoma is a bone lesion.

 A40   (a) True.
(b) True.
(c) True.
(d) False.
(e) True.

Emphysematous inflammation is due to gas-forming organisms and commonest in diabetic patients (due to glucose fermentation). Air is seen tracking on plain film along soft tissue and muscle planes.

Section 5

Obstetrics and gynaecology

Q1 Are the following statements regarding ultrasound of the genital tract true or false?

(a) The uterus and cervix demonstrate different echogenicity.

(b) In the infant the cervix occupies one-third of the uterine length.

(c) In the adult the ovarian volume may be up to 20 ml.

(d) Endometrial thickness in menopausal women on hormone replacement therapy (HRT) may be up to 20 mm.

(e) The Graafian (or dominant) follicle enlarges to 25 mm by day 14 of the menstrual cycle.

Q2 Are the following statements regarding magnetic resonance imaging (MRI) of the uterus true or false?

(a) The junctional zone demonstrates low signal on T2-weighted images.

(b) The endometrium has high signal on T2-weighted images.

(c) Fibroids are usually iso- or hyperintense on T1-weighted images.

(d) Vaginal carcinoma is hyperintense on T2-weighted images.

(e) Uterine adenomyosis is hypointense on T1-weighted images.

(Q3)   Are the following statements regarding ovarian masses true or false?

(a)   Ovarian teratomas are usually solid.
(b)   Ovarian fibromas typically measure 5–10 cm in diameter.
(c)   Teratomas may contain gonadal tissue.
(d)   Brenner's tumours are often cystic.
(e)   Fibromas are associated with weight loss and ascites.

(Q4)   Are the following statements regarding cystic ovarian lesions true or false?

(a)   Cyst walls greater than 1 mm thick have a high likelihood of malignancy.
(b)   Ovarian malignancy may arise in areas of endometriosis.
(c)   Multiparity is a risk factor for ovarian cancer.
(d)   Intracystic septation is a feature suggesting malignancy.
(e)   Doppler blood flow imaging with increased resistive index suggests malignancy.

(Q5)   Are the following statements regarding cervical cancer true or false?

(a)   Ureteric involvement is seen more frequently in cervical than in endometrial cancer.
(b)   FIGO stage II disease may involve the vagina.
(c)   Cervical cancer is the commonest gynaecological malignancy.
(d)   Blurring and widening of the uterine junctional zone are recognised features.
(e)   On T1 the mass lesion appears hypointense.

Are the following statements regarding endometrial cancer true or false?

(a) Tamoxifen use is associated with an increased incidence of endometrial cancer.
(b) Spread to the broad ligaments usually occurs late in the disease.
(c) Ultrasound is usually adequate to stage disease.
(d) An endometrial thickness <5 mm almost always indicates a non-malignant cause of bleeding.
(e) On T2-weighted images, endometrial cancer appears as higher signal than unaffected endometrium.

 Are the following statements regarding endometriosis true or false?

(a) Marked anteversion or anteflexion of the uterus is associated with endometriosis.
(b) Ovarian disease typically presents with cysts of uniform size and echogenicity.
(c) Amniocentesis is a recognised risk factor for development of endometriosis.
(d) Endometrial deposits are typically high signal on T1- and T2-weighted imaging.
(e) Endometrial deposits usually do not enhance with contrast.

 Are the following statements regarding the anatomy of the pelvic ligaments true or false?

(a) The cardinal (transverse cervical) ligament inserts into the piriformis muscle.
(b) The uterosacral ligament arises from the anterior body of the sacrum at S2/S3.
(c) The broad ligament contains the uterine and ovarian arteries.
(d) The median umbilical ligament arises from the trigone of the bladder.

(e) The round ligament attaches to the clitoris via the inguinal canal.

Q9 Are the following statements regarding fibroids true or false?

(a) They may be hypo- or hyperintense relative to the myometrium.
(b) Punctate calcification is particularly seen post partum.
(c) Pedunculated fibroids are significantly more likely to tort during pregnancy.
(d) Braxton Hicks contractions may simulate a fibroid on ultrasound.
(e) Most fibrosarcomas are diagnosed on imaging prior to removal.

Q10 Are the following statements regarding uterine artery embolisation (UAE) for fibroid disease true or false?

(a) Recent uterine sepsis is a contraindication.
(b) Bleeding per vagina (PV) for two to three days post procedure is a recognised side effect.
(c) A general anaesthetic is usually required.
(d) Unilateral UAE has been shown to significantly reduce symptoms.
(e) Pedunculated subserous fibroids are amenable to treatment with UAE.

Q11 Are the following statements regarding polycystic ovarian syndrome (PCOS) true or false?

(a) Polycystic ovaries are seen in approximately 5% of normal women.
(b) The ovaries are usually of normal volume.
(c) The ovarian stroma is generally decreased in echogenicity.
(d) Multiple small cysts are typically scattered peripherally through the ovary.
(e) The degree of hormonal disorder is related to the size and number of ovarian cysts.

Are the following statements regarding malformations of the uterus true or false?

(a) Unicornuate uterus is associated with contralateral renal agenesis.
(b) Uterus bicornis bicollis shows complete uterine division to the internal cervical os.
(c) An intercornual distance of >2 cm implies a bicornuate uterus.
(d) Bicornuate uterus is the commonest uterine anomaly.
(e) Uterus arcuatus shows bilateral abnormally curved uterine horns.

 Are the following statements regarding hysterosalpinography (HSG) (complications/dose) true or false?

(a) A T-shaped uterus is associated with neonatal exposure to warfarin.
(b) Isthmal distension is best achieved in the last 10 days of the menstrual cycle.
(c) Administration of glucagon may be helpful to demonstrate fallopian tube filling.
(d) Non-steroidal anti-inflammatory drugs (NSAIDs) help reduce procedural pain.
(e) Pethidine may be helpful for patients experiencing procedural pain.

(Q14) Are the following statements regarding fetal scanning true or false?

(a) The gestational sac should be visible at 10–14 days' gestation.
(b) Cardiac movement should be detectable by six to seven weeks.
(c) Fetal measurements vary significantly between similar age gestations at 20 weeks.
(d) Crown–rump length is a useful measurement up to 18 weeks.

(e) Fetal parts should be seen with a gestation sac >30 mm diameter.

Q15 Are the following statements regarding gestational tropho-blastic disease true or false?

(a) There is significant variation in the incidence in different countries.
(b) On ultrasound the usual appearance is of an echo poor mass of large cysts.
(c) Fetal parts may be seen.
(d) The serum human chorionic gonadotrophin (hCG) level is not raised in 5–10% of cases.
(e) Of choriocarcinomas, 20–25% are seen following a normal pregnancy.

Q16 Are the following statements regarding the placenta true or false?

(a) Placenta praevia always completely covers the cervical os.
(b) Placenta praevia is commoner in primigravida patients.
(c) Diabetes is a recognised cause of a thickened placenta.
(d) Intrauterine infection is a recognised cause of a thin placenta.
(e) Hyperacute placental abruption is characterised by a hypoechoic area.

Q17 Are the following statements regarding early pregnancy true or false?

(a) Hydronephrosis is a recognised cause of raised serum α-fetoprotein (AFP).
(b) Pleural effusions appear earlier than ascites in fetal heart failure.
(c) Autosomal recessive polycystic kidneys are of increased size with multiple cysts on ultrasound.
(d) Jejunal obstruction demonstrates the double bubble sign.

(e)   Single umbilical vein is associated with an increased incidence of fetal abnormality.

Q18   Are the following statements true or false? After pelvic radiotherapy:

(a)   sacral bone marrow returns increased T1 and T2 signals.
(b)   bladder and rectum return decreased signal on T2.
(c)   the uterus returns increased T2 signal.
(d)   fascial planes generally appear thinned.
(e)   granulation tissue may enhance for years and mimic tumour.

Q19   Are the following statements regarding ectopic pregnancy true or false?

(a)   In vitro fertilisation (IVF) treatment is a recognised risk factor.
(b)   Fifty per cent of cases have normal ultrasound scans.
(c)   Fluid in the pouch of Douglas is a supportive sign.
(d)   Co-existent intra- and extra-uterine pregnancies are seen in 1 in 3 000 000 women.
(e)   A positive pregnancy test may be seen with recent complete abortion.

Q20   Are the following statements regarding the intrauterine contraceptive device (IUCD) true or false?

(a)   A dislodged IUCD may migrate to a subphrenic region.
(b)   Endometritis is usually detectable on ultrasound.
(c)   The Mirena coil is more easily visible on ultrasound than the Lippes loop and Copper 7 devices.
(d)   A correctly positioned IUCD should lie within 10–15 mm of the apex of the fundus.
(e)   Perforation of the uterus by IUCD usually occurs 24–72 hours after the time of insertion.

Answers

 (a) False.
(b) False.
(c) False.
(d) False.
(e) True.

The uterus and cervix demonstrate similar characteristics on ultrasound. In the infant the cervix occupies two-thirds of the uterine length (one-third in the adult). Normal uterine volume is approximately 10 ml. Postmenopausally, normal endometrial thickness is up to 8 mm in women not on HRT, and up to 15 mm in those on HRT.

 (a) True.
(b) True.
(c) False.
(d) False.
(e) False.

Fibroids are iso- or hypointense (due to calcification) on T1-weighted images. Vaginal carcinoma is isointense on T1- and T2-weighted images. Uterine adenomyosis is iso- or hyperintense on T1-weighted images.

 (a) False.
(b) True.
(c) False.
(d) False.
(e) True.

Ovarian teratomas are usually cystic and only occasionally solid. Ovarian fibromas may be large at presentation and have a pedicle which is prone to torsion. Meigs' syndrome consists of weight loss, ascites and a right pleural effusion in combination with an ovarian fibroma. Teratomas may contain all types of tissue except gonadal tissue. Brenner tumours are slow growing, solid, benign masses.

(a) False.
(b) True.
(c) False.
(d) True.
(e) False.

A cut-off value of greater than 3 mm for cyst wall thickness is usually accepted as indicating a higher likelihood of malignancy. Nulliparity is a risk factor for ovarian cancer (as well as age >35 years at time of first child). In an ovarian cyst, the presence of septation, solid elements and mixed echogenicity are features suggestive of malignancy. Doppler blood flow imaging with decreased resistive and pulsatility indices suggests malignancy.

 (a) True.
(b) True.
(c) False.
(d) True.
(e) False.

Ureteric involvement is seen frequently with cervical carcinoma due to the close proximity of the cervix to the ureters and the lesion's propensity to spread to the parametria. FIGO stage II disease may involve the upper two-thirds of the vagina, but extension to the lower third of the vagina or pelvic sidewall constitutes stage III disease. Cervical cancer is the second commonest gynaecological malignancy (after ovarian cancer). Blurring and widening of the uterine junctional zone are recognised features due to the retention of secretions in the uterus from blockage of the cervical canal by tumour. On MRI, the mass lesion appears isointense on T1-weighted images and hyperintense on T2-weighted images.

 (a) True.
(b) True.
(c) False.
(d) True.
(e) False.

Endometrial cancer is associated with: late menarche, polycystic ovarian syndrome, early menopause, obesity, diabetes mellitus, tamoxifen use, oestrogen-only HRT, and oestrogen-secreting ovarian tumours. Spread outside the uterus to the pelvic sidewalls and broad ligaments usually occurs late in the disease. Although ultrasound is sensitive for detecting the primary disease, staging of the pelvis requires MRI. On T2-weighted images, endometrial cancer appears as lower signal than unaffected endometrium and higher signal than myometrium.

A7
(a) False.
(b) False.
(c) True.
(d) True.
(e) False.

Scarring and tethering due to endometriosis usually occur posteriorly, causing uterine retroversion or retroflexion. Ovarian disease typically presents with cysts at different stages of evolution and therefore of differing size and echogenicity. Recognised risk factors for development of endometriosis include uterine surgery and amniocentesis. However, most cases are idiopathic and are thought to be due to peritoneal implantation of endometrial cells via retrograde menstruation or from metaplastic transformation of peritoneal epithelium.

A8
(a) False.
(b) True.
(c) True.
(d) False.
(e) False.

The cardinal (transverse cervical) ligament arises from the cervix and vagina and inserts into the obturator internus muscle. The broad ligament also contains the round and ovarian ligaments. The median umbilical ligament arises from the dome of the bladder and inserts into the umbilicus. The round ligament attaches to the labia majora via the inguinal canal.

A9
(a) True.
(b) False.
(c) True.
(d) True.
(e) False.

Fibroids may be hypo-, iso- or hyperintense relative to the myometrium. Circumferential calcification is seen particularly post partum, with punctate or mulberry calcification seen post menopausally. Fibroids are more likely to necrose (or tort if pedunculated) during pregnancy. The majority of fibrosarcomas are diagnosed on histopathological examination after removal.

(a)   True.
(b)   False.
(c)   False.
(d)   True.
(e)   False.

Recent uterine sepsis is a contraindication, as it makes infection more likely, and severe uterine sepsis may necessitate subsequent hysterectomy. Patients may experience a thin, watery PV discharge for 7–10 days post embolisation. The procedure is performed under local anaesthetic and intravenous analgesia with or without sedation. Unilateral UAE has been shown to significantly reduce symptoms (contrary to previous opinion). Pedunculated subserous fibroids may undergo necrosis and separate from the uterus post embolisation and thus are a relative contraindication to UAE.

(a)   False.
(b)   False.
(c)   False.
(d)   True.
(e)   False.

Polycystic ovaries are seen in approximately 20% of normal women and their appearance alone does not constitute PCOS, which is primarily characterised by hormonal disturbance. The volume of the ovaries usually increases two- to fourfold. The ovarian stroma is generally increased in echogenicity (usually to the same degree as the myometrium, which is usually brighter than the ovarian stroma). Cysts may be either scattered throughout the ovary or arranged peripherally (rosette pattern). The degree of hormonal disorder is unrelated to the size and number of ovarian cysts.

(a) False.
(b) True.
(c) False.
(d) False.
(e) False.

Unicornuate uterus is associated with ipsilateral renal agenesis, uterus didelphys is associated with complete renal agenesis. Uterus bicornis bicollis shows complete uterine division to the internal cervical os (bicornis unicollis is a less extreme form). An intercornual distance of >4 cm or an intercornual angle of 75–105 degrees implies a bicornuate uterus. Septate uterus is the commonest uterine anomaly associated with infertility, uterus arcuatus (in which there is a single abnormally curved uterine horn) is the commonest anomaly not associated with infertility.

 (a) False.
(b) False.
(c) True.
(d) True.
(e) False.

A T-shaped uterus is associated with neonatal exposure to diethylstilbestrol. The first 10 days of the cycle is the best time for HSG because an early pregnancy is extremely unlikely and isthmal distension and tubal filling occur more readily. Some operators routinely prescribe NSAIDs to reduce procedural pain. Pethidine and morphia are contraindicated during the procedure as they stimulate smooth muscle contraction and thus hinder tubal filling.

 (a) False.
(b) True.
(c) False.
(d) False.
(e) True.

The gestational sac is usually visible by 32–35 days' gestation. Cardiac movement should be detectable by six to seven weeks. Fetal measurements do not vary significantly between similar age gestations until after approximately 22 weeks. Crown–rump length is a useful measurement until approximately 10 weeks. Fetal parts should be seen with a gestation sac >30 mm diameter.

(A15)   (a) True.
     (b) False.
     (c) True.
     (d) False.
     (e) True.

There is marked geographic variation in gestational trophoblastic disease with an incidence of 1:2000 pregnancies in Indonesia and 1:1500 in the USA. On ultrasound the usual appearance is of an echogenic mass of small (<15 mm) cysts. Fetal parts may be seen in a partial mole. The serum hCG is invariably raised. Fifty per cent of choriocarcinomas are associated with a molar pregnancy, 25% follow abortion, 22% follow a normal pregnancy and 3% follow an ectopic pregnancy.

(A16)   (a) True.
     (b) False.
     (c) True.
     (d) False.
     (e) False.

By definition, placenta praevia always completely covers the cervical os (otherwise the placenta is termed low-lying). Placenta praevia is commoner in multiparous and older patients and those with previous uterine surgery. Diabetes, intrauterine infection, fetal hydrops, triploidy and rhesus isoimmunisation are recognised causes of a thickened placenta. Intrauterine growth retardation is a recognised cause of a thin placenta. Placental abruption is initially characterised by a hyperechoic area that becomes echo free after one to two weeks.

(a) True.
(b) True.
(c) True.
(d) False.
(e) False.

There are multiple causes of raised serum AFP, including wrong dates, missed abortion, central nervous system and renal anomalies, and anterior body wall defects. Ascites and pericardial effusions appear earlier than pleural effusions in fetal heart failure. Autosomal recessive polycystic kidneys are of increased size and echogenicity on ultrasound (cysts are not visible on ultrasound). Duodenal obstruction demonstrates the double bubble sign; jejunal obstruction demonstrates multiple filled bowel loops. A single umbilical artery is associated with an increased incidence of fetal abnormality (a single umbilical vein is normal).

 (a) True.
(b) False.
(c) False.
(d) False.
(e) True.

After radiotherapy, the sacral bone marrow returns increased T1 and T2 signals (due to fatty conversion of the marrow), the bladder and rectum return increased signal on T2 due to increased vascularity, and the uterus returns decreased T2 signal due to atrophy. Fascial planes are generally thickened.

 (a) True.
(b) False.
(c) True.
(d) False.
(e) True.

Recognised risk factors for ectopic pregnancy include IVF treatment, previous ectopic pregnancy, history of pelvic inflammatory disease or tubal surgery, and IUCD. Twenty per cent of patients with ectopic pregnancy have normal ultrasound scans. Positive supporting signs on ultrasound include endometrial thickening, fluid in the pouch of Douglas and complex adnexal mass. Co-existent intra- and extra-uterine pregnancies are seen in 1 in 30 000 women, rising to 1 in 7000 after induction of ovulation.

 (a) True.
(b) False.
(c) False.
(d) True.
(e) False.

Perforation of the uterus by IUCD usually occurs immediately at the time of insertion and migration may occur anywhere within the abdomen. If the IUCD is not seen within the uterus then an abdominal radiograph is indicated to locate it. Endometritis is usually occult on ultrasound but may manifest as thickening or irregularity of the endometrium. Despite its high efficacy in treating menorrhagia, the Mirena coil has the disadvantage of not being easily visible on ultrasound, particularly in comparison to the older IUCDs.

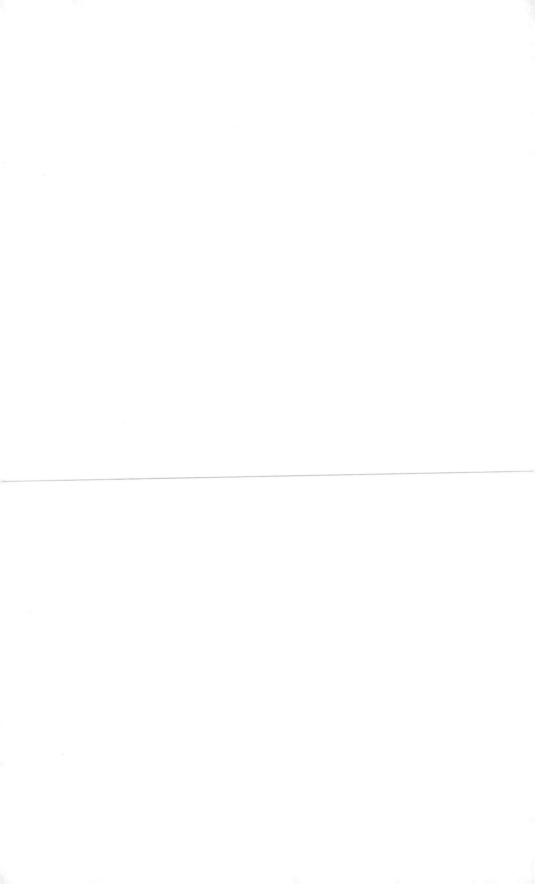

Section 6

Paediatrics

Q1 The following are causes of leukocoria in a child. True or false?

(a) Coat's disease.
(b) Retinopathy of prematurity.
(c) Coloboma.
(d) Neuroblastoma.
(e) Dermoid.

Q2 The following conditions affect the inner ear. True or false?

(a) Mirizzi's syndrome.
(b) Mondini malformation.
(c) Large vestibular aqueduct syndrome.
(d) Cholesteatoma.
(e) Auditory canal atresia.

Q3 Are the following statements regarding ultrasound of the brain and spinal cord in a neonate true or false?

(a) It is commonly performed through the posterior fontanelle.
(b) Grade II intracranial haemorrhage implies ventricular dilatation.
(c) TORCH infections may cause subependymal cysts.
(d) At birth, the conus medullaris lies at the level of the L2/L3 vertebrae in 98% of cases.
(e) The central echo complex is a normal variant in the distal spinal cord.

Q4 Are the following statements regarding scoliosis true or false?

(a) A left thoracic curvature is commoner in idiopathic scoliosis.
(b) The crankshaft phenomenon describes continued spinal deformity due to anterior growth, despite posterior fusion.
(c) May be caused by osteoid osteoma.
(d) The Risser staging system is useful in evaluation.
(e) Patients with Marfan's syndrome are typically affected.

Q5 Are the following statements regarding the paediatric liver true or false?

(a) Focal nodular hyperplasia is a common diagnosis.
(b) Bile duct dilatation is seen in chronic granulomatous disease.
(c) Hepatoblastoma is rarely calcified.
(d) The lesser omentum is thickened in portal hypertension.
(e) Epidermoid cysts of the spleen are usually multilocular.

Q6 The following cause interstitial lung disease in children. True or false?

(a) Respiratory distress syndrome (RDS).
(b) Congenital lymphangiectasia.
(c) Pulmonary haemorrhage.
(d) Cytomegalovirus infection.
(e) Pulmonary atresia.

Q7 The following are associated with Chiari II malformation. True or false?

(a) Lacunar skull.
(b) Beaked tectum of midbrain.
(c) Cerebral heterotopia.
(d) Colpocephaly.
(e) Holoprosencephaly.

Q8   The following conditions may result in dumb-bell shaped bones. True or false?

(a) Osteogenesis imperfecta.
(b) Ellis–van Creveld syndrome.
(c) Mucopolysaccharidoses.
(d) Hypophosphatasia.
(e) Rhabdomyosarcoma.

Q9   Are the following statements regarding small bowel atresia true or false?

(a) The small bowel is the commonest location for gastro-intestinal atresia.
(b) Small bowel stenosis is commoner than atresia.
(c) The patient may pass meconium.
(d) It may be associated with malrotation.
(e) An inherited form is associated with intraluminal calcification.

Q10   The following are causes of pneumatosis intestinalis in infancy. True or false?

(a) Bronchopulmonary dysplasia.
(b) Iron ingestion.
(c) Hypertrophic pyloric stenosis.
(d) Neuroblastoma.
(e) Ascites.

Q11   A hyperlucent lung may be due to the following causes. True or false?

(a) Pulmonary hypogenetic syndrome.
(b) Congenital lobar emphysema.
(c) Pulmonary interstitial emphysema.
(d) Poland's syndrome.
(e) Congenital cyst of the lung.

(Q12)   Are the following statements regarding paediatric fractures true or false?

(a)   Shoulder dislocation is commoner than humeral fractures.
(b)   Clavicular fractures are rare.
(c)   Salter–Harris II are encountered in 75% of epiphyseal injuries.
(d)   The medial humeral condyle is more commonly injured than the lateral condyle.
(e)   Scaphoid fractures are very rare below the age of 10 years.

(Q13)   Soft-tissue abnormalities show the following imaging characteristics. True or false?

(a)   Subcutaneous fat necrosis may cause soft-tissue calcification.
(b)   Haemangiomas are the commonest paediatric soft-tissue tumours.
(c)   Most childhood lipomatous lesions occur in the anterior arm.
(d)   Congenital rhabdomyosarcoma is the commonest malignant lesion in children under 1 year of age.
(e)   Alveolar rhabdomyosarcoma has a good prognosis.

(Q14)   Are the following statements regarding non-accidental injury (NAI) true or false?

(a)   Occipital fractures are more common in NAI than accidental injury.
(b)   Multicystic encephalomalacia is a complication of head injury.
(c)   Scapular fractures are non-specific for NAI.
(d)   The incidence of clavicular fractures is 50%.
(e)   Pancreatic pseudocyst is a recognised feature.

Q15   The following are causes of increased renal reflectivity on ultrasound in neonates. True or false?

(a)   Acute tubular necrosis (ATN).
(b)   Renal vein thrombosis.
(c)   Autosomal recessive polycystic disease.
(d)   Renal dysplasia.
(e)   Neurofibromatosis.

Q16   Are the following statements regarding ultrasound features of Wilm's tumour true or false?

(a)   Calcification is common.
(b)   Classically, there are echo poor regions corresponding to necrosis.
(c)   Stage V implies lung metastases.
(d)   It is associated with duplex kidneys.
(e)   The central sinus echoes are displaced in the precursor, namely nephroblastomatosis.

Q17   Are the following statements regarding neonatal pneumonia true or false?

(a)   Group B streptococci are the commonest cause.
(b)   May be acquired *in utero*.
(c)   Pleural effusions are common.
(d)   It may cause pneumomediastinum.
(e)   Cardiomegaly may occur.

Q18   Are the following statements regarding dextro-transposition true or false?

(a)   It is characterised by ventriculoarterial discordance and atrioventricular concordance.
(b)   The classic plain film appearance is 'egg on side'.
(c)   It is due to faulty cleavage of the bulbus cordis.
(d)   It is more common in females.
(e)   It results in acyanotic congenital heart disease.

Q19   Are the following statements regarding myelination of the paediatric brain true or false?

(a) It begins *in utero*.
(b) It typically begins centrally.
(c) Myelinated areas appear low signal on T2-weighted images.
(d) Leukodystrophies affect grey matter.
(e) Mitochondrial disorders affect both grey and white matter.

Q20   Are the following statements regarding the cervical spine true or false?

(a) The facet joints are more horizontal than in the lumbar spine.
(b) Most movement occurs at C5/C6 level.
(c) Fractures are common relative to thoracic and lumbar spine.
(d) Odontoid peg views are routinely included.
(e) It assumes an adult pattern at 8 years.

Q21   The following may cause irregular or stippled epiphyses. True or false?

(a) Hypothyroidism.
(b) Prenatal infection.
(c) Warfarin ingestion.
(d) Fetal alcohol syndrome.
(e) Diabetes.

Q22   Are the following statements regarding secondary malignancy in children true or false?

(a) It may be genetic or treatment related.
(b) Meningiomas are a common intracranial sequela.
(c) It is dose dependent.
(d) Typically, chondrosarcoma occurs after retinoblastoma treatment.
(e) MRI is preferred to CT for follow-up.

Q23 The following are causes of bowing of the lower limbs. True or false?

(a) Achondroplasia.
(b) Congenital.
(c) Neurofibromatosis.
(d) Hyperthyroidism.
(e) Trauma.

Q24 The following conditions and cardiac lesions are associated. True or false?

(a) Ellis–van Creveld syndrome and atrial septal defect.
(b) Osteogenesis imperfecta and aneurysmal dilatation of the vessels.
(c) Rubella and tricuspid stenosis.
(d) DiGeorge syndrome and interrupted aortic arch.
(e) Fetal alcohol syndrome and patent ductus arteriosus.

Q25 Are the following statements regarding the paediatric oesophagus true or false?

(a) It may give rise to the right main stem bronchus.
(b) Behçet's disease may cause ulceration.
(c) The radiological findings for oesophageal candidiasis are specific.
(d) Graft-versus-host disease may result in web formation.
(e) Mallory–Weiss tears are relatively common.

Q26 Are the following statements true or false?

(a) Cystic hygroma is associated with fetal alcohol syndrome.
(b) The commonest cause of a lesion in the neck is congenital.
(c) Haemophilia is found with enlargement of the epiglottis.
(d) Branchial cysts most commonly arise from the second branchial cleft.

(e)   Normal adenoid tissue becomes visible between 3 and 6 months of age.

Q27   Are the following statements regarding duplication cysts true or false?

(a)   They comprise 1% of all paediatric abdominal masses.
(b)   They are commoner in the oesophagus than the ileum.
(c)   Approximately 50% have co-existent duplication in the gastrointestinal tract.
(d)   They may be associated with duplication of internal genitalia.
(e)   They most often present as a tubular cyst.

Q28   The following conditions are associated. True or false?

(a)   Fibrodysplasia ossificans progressiva and microdactyly of the first toe.
(b)   Homocystinuria and enlarged carpal bones.
(c)   Early osteoarthritis and X-linked spondyloepiphyseal dysplasia.
(d)   Hyperplasia of the radius and Leri–Weill syndrome.
(e)   Trevor's disease and overgrowth of the femoral head epiphysis.

Q29   Are the following statements regarding paediatric ovarian tissue true or false?

(a)   It demonstrates two growth spurts.
(b)   Neonatal cysts may occur.
(c)   Ovarian neoplasms are relatively common.
(d)   It is well vascularised during infancy.
(e)   Ultrasonic features of polycystic ovaries may be visible.

Q30   Are the following statements regarding nephroblastomatosis true or false?

(a)   It is found in 0.1% of infant kidneys.
(b)   It is derived from metanephric blastema normally present up to 36 weeks.

(c) It is only perilobar in location.
(d) It is associated with trisomy 18.
(e) It is hyperintense on T1-weighted MRI.

Answers

 (a) True.
(b) True.
(c) False.
(d) False.
(e) False.

Coat's disease is a congenital vascular anomaly involving the retina, characterised by the presence of leaking ectatic vessels with lipid exudates. It is usually unilateral, is non-calcified and causes retinal detachment. Retinopathy of prematurity is often bilateral and shows dense retrolental membranes and extensive retinal detachment. Coloboma arises from a defect in closure of the optic fissure in the embryo resulting in micro-ophthalmia and a peripheral defect in the globe. Retinoblastoma typically causes leukocoria. Dermoid tumours are extra-ocular and occur along lines of embryonic closure, such as that adjacent to the lateral canthus of the eye.

 (a) False.
(b) True.
(c) True.
(d) False.
(e) False.

The following anomalies affect the inner ear: Mondini and Michel malformations, large vestibular aqueduct syndrome and hypoplasia of the internal auditory canal. Mirizzi's syndrome is secondary compression of the common hepatic duct due to a large gallstone at the cystic duct, with chronic inflammation. Cholesteatoma affects the middle ear cavity and auditory canal atresia affects the outer ear.

(a) False.
(b) False.
(c) True.
(d) True.
(e) True.

Ultrasound is commonly performed through the anterior fontanelle. Grade II haemorrhage is intraventricular haemorrhage without ventricular dilatation.

 (a) True.
(b) True.
(c) True.
(d) True.
(e) True.

Osteoid osteoma in the spine may cause a painful scoliosis. The Risser system (grades 0–5) is based on the degree of ossification of the iliac crest apophysis, grade 4 equating to cessation of spinal growth. Up to 75% of Marfan's patients are affected by scoliosis. In a skeletally immature patient, the crankshaft phenomenon occurs when isolated posterior arthrodesis acts as a tethering bar, producing lordosis and bending of the spine as the unfused anterior vertebral bodies continue to grow.

 (a) False.
(b) True.
(c) False.
(d) True.
(e) False.

Focal nodular hyperplasia and adenoma are rare in the paediatric population. Hepatoblastoma is often calcified. Epidermoid cysts of the spleen are usually unilocular.

 (a) True.
(b) True.
(c) True.
(d) True.
(e) False.

RDS (hyaline membrane disease) may cause lobar/interstitial emphysema, or bronchopulmonary dysplasia. Congenital lymphangiectasia is a malformation characterised by anomalous dilatation of pulmonary lymph vessels and is invariably fatal before two months of age. Pulmonary atresia usually comprises an atretic pulmonary valve with underdevelopment of the pulmonary artery. The affected lung is small but otherwise normal initially, although pulmonary hypertension may ensue without treatment.

  (a) True.
         (b) True.
         (c) True.
         (d) True.
         (e) False.

The features of Chiari II malformation are:

- *Skull and dura*: lacunar skull, small posterior fossa, fenestrated falx cerebri, concave clivus, gaping foramen magnum.
- *Brain*: inferior displacement of the vermis, medullary kink, interdigitation of the gyri, towering cerebellum, callosal dysgenesis, heterotopia, polymicrogyria.
- *Ventricles*: hydrocephalus in 90%, elongated fourth ventricle, large massa intermedia, high riding third ventricle, colpocephaly of the lateral ventricles.
- *Spine and cord*: myelomeningocele (100%), syringohydromyelia (50–90%), diastematomyelia, segmentation anomalies (<10%), incomplete arch of C1 vertebra.

  (a) True.
         (b) True.
         (c) False.
         (d) False.
         (e) False.

Osteogenesis imperfecta typically causes expanded proximal humeri and femora, as well as biconcave vertebral bodies. Ellis–van Creveld syndrome (chondroectodermal dysplasia) is a very rare condition causing ectodermal dysplasia (manifested by absent or hypoplastic nails, irregular/pointed teeth, fine/sparse hair) among other abnormalities. If mucopolysaccharidoses affect the bones they tend to cause expansion of the diaphyses with distal tapering. Hypophosphatasia causes a rickets-like syndrome.

 (a) True.
(b) False.
(c) True.
(d) True.
(e) True.

The small bowel is the commonest location for gastrointestinal atresia (1 in 750 live births), with the ileum being affected slightly more often than the jejunum. It is usually due to a prenatal insult affecting the vascular supply. Contrast studies are not generally required for jejunal atresia, however, they are required for ileal atresia to differentiate from other causes of low obstruction. 'Apple-peel' syndrome occurs in less than 5% of cases, where there is absence of the superior mesenteric artery and most of the ileum. The presence of multiple small and large bowel atresias with intraluminal calcification has an autosomal inheritance.

 (a) True.
(b) True.
(c) True.
(d) False.
(e) False.

Other causes include: malrotation and volvulus, steroids, congenital heart disease, short bowel syndrome, viral gastroenteritis, Hirschsprung's disease, neutropenic colitis and cystic fibrosis.

 (a) True.
(b) True.
(c) True.
(d) False.
(e) True.

Pulmonary hypogenetic syndrome comprises a spectrum ranging from hypoplasia to complete agenesis. Pulmonary vascularity in the affected lung is typically diminished. In congenital lobar emphysema the affected lobe is hyperexpanded and thus trans-lucent (once the secretions within it have cleared). Pulmonary interstitial emphysema is a complication of ventilation in which air escapes hyperinflated alveoli into the interstitium and occasion-ally the mediastinum. In Poland's syndrome (congenital absence of the sternocostal head of pectoralis major) the chest (but not the lung itself) is hyperlucent.

 (a) False.
(b) False.
(c) True.
(d) False.
(e) True.

Shoulder dislocation is comparatively unusual in the paediatric group. Clavicular fractures are common. Salter–Harris II are the commonest type of fracture, encountered in 75% of epiphyseal injuries. The lateral humeral condyle is more vulnerable than the medial. Scaphoid fractures are very rare below the age of 10 years, the effecting forces usually causing fracture at the distal radius, humerus or clavicle.

 (a) True.
(b) True.
(c) False.
(d) False.
(e) False.

Most childhood lipomas occur in the posterior thigh. Congenital fibrosarcoma is the commonest soft-tissue malignant lesion below the age of 1 year. Alveolar and undifferentiated rhabdomyosar-comas have a poor prognosis, botryoid and spindle cell rhabdo-myosarcomas have a good prognosis.

 (a) True.
(b) True.
(c) False.
(d) False.
(e) True.

Occipital fractures often result from a blow to the back of the head. Multicystic encephalomalacia is a long-term sequela of head injury and may indicate an old injury. The incidence of clavicular fractures is 2–6%. Scapular fractures are unusual in genuine accidental injuries and are suggestive of NAI. Post-traumatic pancreatic pseudocyst is a recognised feature.

  (a) True.
      (b) True.
      (c) True.
      (d) True.
      (e) False.

	Large kidneys	*Small kidneys*	*Normal kidneys*
C/M preserved	ATN RVT (early) Nephrotic syndrome	Hypoplasia RVT (late)	Normal ATN Septicaemia
C/M loss	RVT ARPKD Congenital nephrosis Storage disorders	Dysplasia	Storage disorders
C/M reversal	ARPKD		

C/M, corticomedullary differentiation; ATN, acute tubular necrosis; RVT, renal vein thrombosis; ARPKD, autosomal recessive polycystic kidney disease.

  (a) False.
      (b) True.
      (c) False.
      (d) True.
      (e) True.

Calcification is uncommon, however, when it occurs, it is denser than neuroblastoma. Stage V implies bilateral renal involvement. Associations include: aniridia, hemihypertrophy, Beckwith–Wiedemann syndrome, and anomalies of the renal (horseshoe

kidney, duplex, solitary or fused kidney) and genital (crypt-
orchidism, hypospadias) systems.

(A17) (a) True.
       (b) True.
       (c) False.
       (d) True.
       (e) True.

Group B streptococci are the commonest cause of neonatal pneumonia, particularly in low-birthweight infants, and has 50% mortality. Other organisms implicated are *Pneumococcus, Listeria,
Candida, Chlamydia, Escherichia coli* and *Pneumocystis*. The
radiological appearances include bilateral focal/diffuse opacification,
hyperaeration, lobar atelectasis and pneumothorax.

(A18) (a) True.
       (b) True.
       (c) True.
       (d) False.
       (e) False.

Dextro-transposition is commoner in males and results in cyanosis.

(A19) (a) True.
       (b) True.
       (c) True.
       (d) False.
       (e) True.

Myelination begins at five months *in utero*, progresses caudally to
cranially, centrally to peripherally and dorsally to ventrally. Leukodystrophies affect white matter.

(A20) (a) True.
       (b) False.
       (c) False.
       (d) False.
       (e) True.

Most movement occurs at C2/C3 and C3/C4. Cervical spine fractures are uncommon and account for less than 2% of spinal injuries.

 (a) True.
(b) True.
(c) True.
(d) True.
(e) False.

Other causes include avascular necrosis, Morquio's syndrome, multiple epiphyseal dysplasia, chondrodysplasia punctata, Zellweger's syndrome and trisomies 18 and 21, and they may be a normal variant.

 (a) True.
(b) True.
(c) True.
(d) False.
(e) True.

Treatment-related malignancy occurs after chemotherapy or radiotherapy. Typically, osteosarcoma occurs after retinoblastoma. MRI is non-ionising and therefore ideal for follow-up.

 (a) True.
(b) True.
(c) True.
(d) False.
(e) True.

Hypothyroidism is a cause of bowing of the lower limbs.

 (a) True.
(b) True.
(c) False.
(d) True.
(e) False.

Ellis–van Creveld syndrome is associated with atrial and ventricular septal defects. Rubella syndrome is associated with patent ductus arteriosus, pulmonary stenosis and hypoplasia. Ventricular septal defect is found in conjunction with fetal alcohol syndrome.

 A25
(a) True.
(b) True.
(c) False.
(d) True.
(e) False.

Behçet's disease may cause ulceration almost anywhere in the gastrointestinal or genitourinary tract. The radiological findings for oesophageal candidiasis are non-specific and the differential includes herpes or cytomegalovirus oesophagitis, caustic ulceration and oesophageal varices. Graft-versus-host disease may result in web formation. Mallory–Weiss tears are usually associated with alcohol ingestion and are uncommon in children.

 A26
(a) True.
(b) True.
(c) True.
(d) True.
(e) True.

Cystic hygroma is associated with fetal alcohol syndrome, and Turner's and Noonan's syndromes. Fifty-five per cent of lesions in the paediatric neck are congenital, the less common causes being inflammation (27%) and malignancy (11%).

 A27
(a) False.
(b) False.
(c) False.
(d) True.
(e) False.

Duplication cysts comprise 15% of all paediatric abdominal masses and are most commonly found in the ileum, then oesophagus, colon and jejunum; 10–15% have coexistent duplication in the gastrointestinal tract. They usually present as a spherical cyst and less commonly as a tubular cyst.

(a) True.
(b) True.
(c) True.
(d) False.
(e) True.

Hypoplasia of the radius (Madelung's deformity) is associated with Leri–Weill disease, which is typically bilateral and results in limited motion of the elbow and wrist (autosomal dominant inheritance).

 (a) True.
(b) True.
(c) False.
(d) False.
(e) True.

The two growth spurts occur at 8 years (adrenarche) and just before puberty. Ovarian neoplasms are very rare (<1%). Ovarian tissue is poorly vascularised in infancy; however, this improves during the growth spurts. Imaging features suggesting polycystic ovarian syndrome are ovarian enlargement, with at least 10 peripherally placed cysts measuring between 2 mm and 8 mm.

 (a) False.
(b) True.
(c) False.
(d) True.
(e) False.

Nephroblastomatosis may be both perilobar and intralobar and is found in 0.1% of infant kidneys. There are multiple associations including Beckwith–Weidemann syndrome, hemihypertrophy, trisomy 18 and Perlman's syndrome. It is hypointense on T1-weighted MRI.

Section 7

Central nervous system

Q1 Are the following statements regarding herpes simplex encephalitis true or false?

(a) Computed tomography (CT) scan is often negative for the first week.

(b) The putamen is normally spared.

(c) Haemorrhage is rarely seen.

(d) The frontal lobes are more commonly affected than the temporal lobes.

(e) Imaging changes are usually bilateral.

Q2 Are the following statements regarding extra-dural (epi-dural) haematomas true or false?

(a) Extra-dural (epidural) haematomas may cross suture lines.

(b) A skull fracture is associated with 75–95% of extra-dural haematomas.

(c) More than 50% of patients have a lucid interval.

(d) Disruption of dural sinuses is a common cause in young children.

(e) The attenuation of fresh blood is approximately 50–80 Hounsfield units (HU).

Q3 Are the following statements regarding intracerebral haem-atoma on magnetic resonance imaging (MRI) true or false?

(a) Fresh bleeding (<1 hour) is isointense on T1.

(b) At one to three days the haematoma is predominantly hypointense on T1.
(c) At three to seven days the haematoma is hyperintense on T1.
(d) At 8–14 days the haematoma is hypointense on T2.
(e) At 14–21 days the haematoma is bright on T1.

Q4 Are the following statements regarding hypothalamic hamartoma true or false?

(a) It is associated with attacks of laughing.
(b) Its appearance on imaging remains stable over time.
(c) It is usually not located within the hypothalamus.
(d) It enhances on CT with intravenous contrast.
(e) It is isointense on T1 MRI.

Q5 Are the following statements regarding carotid artery dissection true or false?

(a) The accuracy of ultrasound assessment is 60–80%.
(b) Smoking is a recognised risk factor.
(c) An intimal flap is seen on angiography in 50–70% of patients.
(d) On MRI the affected artery often appears enlarged.
(e) The commonest level affected is C5–C7.

Q6 Are the following statements regarding choroid plexus papilloma true or false?

(a) Peak age is between six and 10 years.
(b) The commonest location is within the third ventricle.
(c) It may transform into choroid plexus carcinoma.
(d) Calcification is rare.
(e) The ventricles typically appear asymmetrically dilated.

Q7 Are the following statements regarding haemangioblastomas of the neuraxis true or false?

(a) There is a recognised association with tuberous sclerosis.

(b) They are commoner in the spinal cord than the cerebellum.
(c) Angiography may be indicated before surgery.
(d) About 1–2% present as solid lesions.
(e) Spinal haemangioblastomas are commonly associated with syringomyelia.

Q8 Are the following statements regarding the internal carotid artery (ICA) and its branches true or false?

(a) The ophthalmic artery is the first branch as the ICA leaves the cavernous sinus.
(b) The cervical portion of the ICA has no branches.
(c) The ICA passes through the anterior part of the foramen lacerum.
(d) The ICA ascends posterolateral to the external carotid artery.
(e) The ICA ascends lateral to the anterior clinoid processes.

Q9 Are the following statements regarding cerebrospinal fluid (CSF) true or false?

(a) Total volume of CSF in an adult is approximately 500 ml.
(b) It is exclusively formed by the choroid plexuses.
(c) Most of the CSF flows superolaterally over the cerebral hemispheres.
(d) It flows from the fourth ventricle anteriorly via the foramen of Magendie.
(e) Flow within the cerebral aqueduct is pulsatile.

Q10 Are the following statements regarding magnetic resonance angiography (MRA) true or false?

(a) In time of flight (TOF) MRA, flowing blood demonstrates high signal.
(b) Intravenous contrast is required for phase contrast MRA.

(c) Pre-saturation pulses are helpful for distinguishing arteries and veins in phase contrast MRA.
(d) TOF MRA is usually quicker than phase contrast MRA.
(e) Phase contrast MRA is quantitative.

Q11 Are the following statements regarding cerebral HIV/AIDS true or false?

(a) If only a single lesion is present then toxoplasmosis is less likely than lymphoma.
(b) Cytomegalovirus typically presents with cognitive dysfunction.
(c) Hydrocephalus is a recognised presentation of crypto-coccosis.
(d) Progressive multifocal leukoencephalopathy (PML) lesions are usually diffuse and symmetrical.
(e) Toxoplasmosis lesions commonly occur in the basal ganglia.

Q12 Are the following statements regarding pituitary tumours true or false?

(a) Prolactin secretion correlates well with tumour size.
(b) Most pituitary tumours are greater than 1 cm at presentation.
(c) Prolactin-secreting tumours are equally common in men and women.
(d) Pituitary adenomas are usually high signal on T2-weighted MRI.
(e) Corticotrophic adenomas usually arise from the anterior lobe of the pituitary.

Q13 Are the following statements regarding tuberous sclerosis true or false?

(a) Tuber calcifications do not progress after birth.
(b) Giant cell astrocytomas of the fourth ventricle are a recognised complication.

(c) Grey matter heterotopia appears as hyperintensity on T1-weighted MRI.
(d) Cortical tubers are only rarely bilateral.
(e) Subependymal hamartomas may line the third and fourth ventricles.

(Q14) Are the following statements regarding neurofibromatosis true or false?

(a) Neurofibromatosis type 1 is associated with bilateral acoustic neuromas.
(b) Neurofibromatosis type 1 is associated with optic nerve gliomas in 20–30% of patients.
(c) Multiple T1 bright lesions are a recognised feature.
(d) Benign aqueductal stenosis causing hydrocephalus is a recognised feature.
(e) Plexiform neurofibromas usually present at the foramen magnum.

(Q15) Are the following statements regarding cerebral malformations true or false?

(a) Lissencephaly presents with an abnormally thick grey matter.
(b) In incomplete lissencephaly the frontal lobes are most commonly affected.
(c) Polymicrogyria presents with thinned cortex.
(d) In open lip schizencephaly white matter lines the cleft.
(e) Schizencephaly is most commonly bilateral.

(Q16) Are the following statements regarding imaging in epilepsy true or false?

(a) Hippocampal sclerosis is best assessed on fine-cut axial T2 MR images.
(b) Hippocampal sclerosis is associated with ipsilateral atrophy of the fornix.
(c) Areas of cortical dysplasia usually have a small amount of mass effect.

(d) Juvenile myoclonic epilepsy usually shows no abnormality on conventional imaging.

(e) Cerebral cavernous haemangiomas often present with epilepsy.

Q17 Are the following statements regarding neurocysticercosis true or false?

(a) The infestation arises from beef tapeworms.

(b) The meninges are more commonly affected than the brain parenchyma.

(c) Focal calcifications do not appear for at least two years.

(d) Living larvae are visualised as areas with associated oedema.

(e) The white matter may appear generally oedematous.

Q18 Are the following statements regarding Dandy–Walker malformation (DWM) true or false?

(a) DWM is characterised by dilatation of the third ventricle.

(b) DWM is associated with midline cerebral anomalies.

(c) On imaging, the torcular herophili lies superior to the lambdoid angle.

(d) DWM is associated with syndactyly.

(e) Dandy–Walker variant syndrome is associated with posterior fossa enlargement.

Q19 Are the following statements regarding cerebral arteriovenous malformations (AVM) true or false?

(a) Affected arteries have relatively thickened elastic walls.

(b) AVM may present with progressive neurological deficit.

(c) Thrombosed AVMs typically fail to enhance with contrast.

(d) Negative angiography is a recognised finding.

(e)   Calcification is seen on skull radiographs in 10–20%
of cases.

Q20   Are the following statements regarding diffuse axonal injury true or false?

(a)   It is typical of rotational injury.
(b)   Lesions are typically based in the deep white matter.
(c)   Lesions in the corpus callosum are usually anterior.
(d)   The medulla is often affected.
(e)   CT is more sensitive than MRI for lesion detection.

Q21   Are the following statements regarding multiple sclerosis
(MS) and demyelination true or false?

(a)   White matter lesions in the corpus callosum are highly
specific for MS.
(b)   T1-weighted images are more sensitive for white matter lesions than fluid attenuated inversion recovery
(FLAIR) images.
(c)   Lesions in the spinal cord are seen in 10–20% of cases
of MS.
(d)   White matter lesions are typically orientated medio-
laterally.
(e)   In acute disseminated encephalomyelitis (ADEM) both
grey and white matter lesions may be seen.

Q22   Are the following statements regarding cerebral anatomy
true or false?

(a)   The foramen rotundum transmits the mandibular nerve.
(b)   The foramen spinosum is anteromedial to the foramen
ovale.
(c)   The foramen ovale transmits the middle meningeal
artery.
(d)   The foramen ovale is posterolateral to the foramen
rotundum.
(e)   The foramen lacerum is located at the base of the
lateral pterygoid plate.

Q23   Are the following statements regarding meningioma true or false?

(a)   Meningioma is the commonest benign intracranial tumour.
(b)   It commonly presents with bony erosion.
(c)   It is usually hypointense on T1-weighted MRI.
(d)   Small tumours typically have an internal and external carotid blood supply.
(e)   It may present as focal expansion of the paranasal sinuses.

Q24   Are the following statements regarding posterior cranial fossa tumours true or false?

(a)   The majority of adult intracranial tumours arise in the posterior fossa.
(b)   The incidence of medulloblastoma peaks in the second and third decades.
(c)   Approximately 50% of medulloblastomas calcify.
(d)   Medulloblastomas typically enhance uniformly.
(e)   Ependymomas are usually located in the roof of the fourth ventricle.

Q25   Are the following statements regarding cerebral metastases true or false?

(a)   They can be well visualised using fluorodeoxyglucose positron emission tomography (FDG-PET).
(b)   They typically occur deep in the white matter.
(c)   Metastases from malignant melanomas are typically high signal on T1 and T2 imaging.
(d)   Metastases from chondrosarcomas may ossify.
(e)   They typically demonstrate irregular, shaggy enhancement with contrast.

Answers

 A1 (a) False.
(b) True.
(c) False.
(d) False.
(e) False.

Herpes simplex encephalitis is the commonest form of non-epidemic meningoencephalitis in the western world. Magnetic resonance imaging (MRI) is usually more sensitive than CT, demonstrating increased signal on T2. The role of CT (which may be negative for the first three days) is mainly to identify a biopsy site. Changes of decreased attenuation (often with areas of haemorrhage) are usually unilateral with the temporal lobes affected more commonly than the frontal and parietal lobes. The putamen is typically spared, thus forming a sharply defined straight or concave border.

 A2 (a) True.
(b) True.
(c) False.
(d) True.
(e) False.

Extra-dural haematomas are present in 2% of serious head injuries and arise between the inner table of the skull and the calvarial periosteum, a dural layer which is bound down at the suture margins. The only circumstance under which they may cross suture lines is when there is a diastatic suture fracture. For example, in children when a diastatic fracture of the lambdoid and coronal suture is associated with a tear of the sagittal and transverse venous sinuses. Between 75% and 95% are associated with a skull fracture (less commonly in children). Attenuation of fresh extravasated blood is 30–50 HU and coagulated blood 50–80 HU. Fewer than 33% of patients have a lucid interval.

 A3 (a) True.
(b) True.
(c) True.

(d) False.
(e) False.

Hyperacute haemorrhage (<1 hour) is isointense on T1 and hyper-intense on T2. Deoxygenation of the haemoglobin then occurs and between one and three days an acute haematoma is typically hypointense on T1 and T2. Then oxidation occurs and at three to seven days the intracellular methaemoglobin in the early sub-acute haematoma is hyperintense on T1 and hypointense on T2. At 8–14 days the late subacute haematoma is hyperintense on T1 and T2 due to the presence of extracellular methaemoglobin. From the fourteenth day onwards haemosiderin is present, which is hypo-intense on T1 and T2.

  (a) True.
(b) True.
(c) True.
(d) False.
(e) True.

Hypothalamic hamartoma is a congenital malformation asso-ciated with gelastic seizures (uncontrollable attacks of laughing). It is composed of a collection of heterotopic normal neuronal tissue located at or close to the mamillary bodies and is only rarely found within the hypothalamus itself. On CT and MRI it is isointense with brain tissue and does not enhance with intravenous contrast.

  (a) False.
(b) True.
(c) False.
(d) True.
(e) False.

Ultrasound is relatively inaccurate, only diagnosing carotid artery dissection in about 50% of patients. MRI is more accurate and usually demonstrates apparent enlargement of the vessel due to intramural haematoma. Angiography is the gold standard and typically demonstrates a 'string sign', i.e. a long segment of tapered luminal narrowing extending up to the skull base. An intimal flap is only seen in approximately 30% of patients. The commonest level affected is C1–C2. Risk factors include hypertension, smoking, migraine and trauma.

 (a) False.
(b) False.
(c) True.
(d) False.
(e) True.

Choroid plexus papilloma represents up to 5% of childhood brain tumours and more than 80% present before the age of five years. They are most commonly located within the trigone of the lateral ventricles and less commonly within the third or fourth ventricles. Cerebrospinal fluid overproduction or obstruction typically causes asymmetrically dilated ventricles. They may transform into carcinoma and the two tumours are radiographically similar. They commonly undergo calcification.

 (a) False.
(b) False.
(c) True.
(d) False.
(e) True.

Haemangioblastomas of the neuraxis are benign tumours of vascular origin, commonest in the cerebellum (80%) and are associated with von Hippel–Lindau disease. Although typically presenting as cysts with or without a mural nodule, 10–30% present as solid lesions. Angiography is often indicated before surgery to identify the vascular supply and drainage. Spinal haemangioblastomas are associated with syringomyelia in 70% of cases.

 (a) True.
(b) True.
(c) False.
(d) False.
(e) False.

The cervical portion of the ICA has no branches and ascends posteromedial to the external carotid artery. In its petrous segment it passes through the anterior portion of the foramen lacerum to the cavernous sinus. It exits the cavernous sinus medial to the anterior clinoid processes and the ophthalmic artery is the first major branch.

 (a) False.
(b) False.
(c) True.
(d) True.
(e) True.

Although the amount of CSF producted per day is 500 ml, the circulating volume in an adult is about 150 ml. It is mainly formed by choroid plexuses, but some CSF is formed by the neural paren-chyma. Most of the CSF flows superolaterally over the cerebral hemispheres. From the lateral ventricles it flows via the foramen of Monro to the third ventricle. It passes from the third ventricle with pulsatile flow via the cerebral aqueduct to the fourth ventricle, from where it exits laterally via the foramina of Luschka and posteromedially via the foramen of Magendie.

 (a) True.
(b) False.
(c) False.
(d) True.
(e) True.

In TOF imaging repetitive excitations decrease the magnetisation of the blood within the sample volume: blood flowing in will still be magnetised and thus appears of high signal. Since arteries and veins on opposite sides of the sample volume will contribute fully mag-netised blood, a pre-saturation pulse is applied on one side of the volume to demagnetise blood there and thus select only arterial blood from one direction. TOF imaging is usually quicker than phase contrast (approximately 60 seconds versus 200 seconds). Phase contrast MRA relies on calculating the difference between signals from voxels using velocity-insensitive and velocity-sensitive sequences: the net result is the velocity vector. Although quanti-tative, the technique is time consuming. Contrast-enhanced MRA is also available and is quicker than phase contrast or TOF MRA.

(a) False.
(b) True.
(c) True.
(d) False.
(e) True.

If only a single lesion is present then toxoplasmosis and lymphoma are equally likely; if multiple lesions are present toxoplasmosis is more likely. In the immunocompromised patient hydrocephalus is a recognised presentation of cryptococcosis. PML lesions are typically well defined and asymmetrical.

 (a) False.
(b) True.
(c) False.
(d) True.
(e) False.

Prolactin secretion correlates poorly with tumour size. Prolactin-secreting tumours are less common in men than women (unlike macroadenomas which are usually non-secreting and equally common in men and women). Pituitary adenomas are usually high signal on T2-weighted MRI, and low signal on T1. Corticotrophic adenomas usually arise from the posterior lobe of the pituitary.

 (a) False.
(b) False.
(c) False.
(d) False.
(e) True.

Tuber calcifications progress with age. Giant cell astrocytomas are seen at the foramen of Monro where they may cause obstructive hydrocephalus. Grey matter heterotopic areas present as subtle T1 hypointensities and well-defined T2 hyperintensities. In 30–40% of cases cortical tubers are bilateral.

 (a) False.
(b) True.
(c) False.

(d) True.
(e) False.

Neurofibromatosis type 2 is associated with bilateral acoustic neuromas. Multiple T1 isointense and T2 hyperintense lesions are thought to reflect areas of dysmyelination. Hydrocephalus may be seen due to benign aqueductal stenosis or glioma. Plexiform neurofibromas usually present at the orbital apex or superior orbital fissure.

 (a) True.
(b) False.
(c) False.
(d) False.
(e) True.

In incomplete lissencephaly the parieto-occipital areas are most commonly affected. Polymicrogyria presents with thickened cortex (but multiple poorly formed gyri). In open lip schizencephaly grey matter lines the cleft.

 (a) False.
(b) True.
(c) False.
(d) True.
(e) True.

Hippocampal sclerosis is usually best assessed on fine-cut coronal MR images. Areas of cortical dysplasia have no mass effect. Cerebral cavernous haemangiomas often present with epilepsy (79–80%).

 (a) False.
(b) True.
(c) False.
(d) False.
(e) True.

The infestation arises from pork tapeworms. The meninges are affected nearly twice as frequently as the brain parenchyma (~40% versus 20%). Focal calcifications may appear within six months.

Larvae elicit oedema when they die. In acute neurocysticercosis the white matter may appear generally oedematous.

 (a) False.
(b) True.
(c) True.
(d) True.
(e) False.

DWM is characterised by dilatation of the fourth ventricle, enlarged posterior fossa (unlike Dandy–Walker variant syndrome) and agenesis of the cerebellar vermis. It is strongly associated with midline cerebral anomalies as well as other malformations such as cleft palate, syndactyly and polydactyly.

 (a) False.
(b) True.
(c) True.
(d) True.
(e) True.

Affected arteries have relatively thinned walls with deficient elastin. Negative angiography is a recognised finding and may be due to thrombosis or compression of the vessels of the AVM by haematoma. Calcification is usually speckled or ring-like.

 (a) True.
(b) False.
(c) False.
(d) False.
(e) False.

Lesions are typically based at the grey/white matter interface and always spare the cortex. Lesions in the corpus callosum are usually mid or posterior. The brainstem and upper pons are often affected. MRI is more sensitive than CT and demonstrates hyperintense foci on T2-weighted imaging.

 (a) True.
(b) False.
(c) True.

(d) False.
(e) True.

White matter lesions in the corpus callosum are highly specific for MS, being rare in others diseases such as cerebrovascular disease. T2-weighted and FLAIR (heavily T2-weighted with bulk fluid suppression) images are more sensitive for white matter lesions than T1 images. Lesions in the spinal cord are seen in 10–20% of cases of MS. White matter lesions are typically orientated antero-posteriorly. The majority of ADEM lesions are in the white matter but grey matter lesions may also be seen.

 (a) False.
(b) False.
(c) False.
(d) True.
(e) False.

These three foramina are orientated in an oblique line, from anteromedially behind the superior orbital fissure to posterolaterally: rotundum, ovale, spinosum. The foramen rotundum transmits the maxillary nerve, the foramen ovale the mandibular nerve and the foramen spinosum the middle meningeal artery. The foramen lacerum is located at the base of the medial pterygoid plate.

 (a) True.
(b) False.
(c) True.
(d) False.
(e) True.

Meningioma is the commonest benign intracranial tumour, representing 15% of all intracranial tumours. It commonly presents with bony hyperostosis and only occasionally with erosion. It is usually iso- or hypointense on T1-weighted MRI, being iso- or slightly hyperintense on T2-weighted and enhances avidly with contrast. Large tumours often have an internal and external carotid blood supply. Several patterns of growth have been described including en plaque, globular, multicentric and pneumosinus dilatans (focal expansion of the paranasal sinuses).

(a) False.
(b) False.
(c) False.
(d) True.
(e) False.

The majority of paediatric intracranial tumours arise in the posterior fossa unlike adult tumours. There are two peaks of incidence of medulloblastoma, in the first decade and in late adulthood. Approximately 10% of medulloblastomas calcify and they typically present in the midline in children and laterally in adults. They are usually well defined and enhance uniformly. Ependymomas are usually located in the floor of the fourth ventricle. They may enhance uniformly or non-uniformly and are calcified in 50% of cases.

 (a) False.
(b) False.
(c) True.
(d) False.
(e) False.

Cerebral metastases are poorly visualised with FDG-PET because of the high background activity. Metastases spread haematogenously and usually lodge at the grey/white matter interface. Metastases from malignant melanomas are typically high signal on T1 and T2 imaging (due to melanin). Metastases from osteosarcomas may ossify. Metastases usually demonstrate regular enhancement; if enhancement is irregular or shaggy, cerebral abscess should be suspected.

Section 8

Dental

Q1 Are the following statements regarding dentigerous cysts true or false?

(a) A dentigerous cyst is invariably associated with an unerupted tooth.

(b) Unerupted teeth are associated with ameloblastomas.

(c) Dentigerous cysts are typically associated with the upper and lower first molars.

(d) Impacted teeth are particularly associated with radicular cysts.

(e) Non-vital teeth are associated with adenomatoid odontogenic tumours.

Q2 Are the following statements regarding cystic lesions in the jaw true or false?

(a) Most ameloblastomas occur in the maxilla.

(b) Nasolabial cysts may cause adjacent maxillary bone resorption.

(c) Multiple periodontal cysts occur in Gorlin's syndrome.

(d) Periapical cysts usually develop in carious teeth.

(e) Hypoparathyroidism may cause cystic lesions in the jaw.

Q3 The following are recognised causes of loss of the lamina dura. True or false?

(a) Osteoporosis.

(b) Addison's disease.

(c) Paget's disease.

(d) Scleroderma.
(e) Langerhans cell histiocytosis.

Q4 Are the following statements regarding the jaw true or false?

(a) The inferior alveolar nerve exits the mandible via the mandibular foramen.
(b) The temporalis muscle is innervated by the maxillary branch of the trigeminal nerve.
(c) Computed tomography (CT) scan is indicated to assess the alveolar process anatomy before placement of dental implants.
(d) Mandibular fractures tend to be orientated perpendicular to the long axis of the roots of the teeth.
(e) Taste fibres from the anterior two-thirds of the tongue are carried in the chorda tympani nerve.

Q5 Are the following statements regarding the jaw true or false?

(a) Diagnosis of mandibular osteomyelitis often requires serial CT scanning.
(b) Unilateral mandibular fractures are commoner than bilateral fractures.
(c) The dose for an orthopantomogram (OPG) is approximately 10–25 mSv.
(d) The dose for a bitewing radiograph is more than for an orthopantomogram.
(e) If a bitewing film needs to be held still this should be done by the patient.

Answers

  (a) True.
(b) True.
(c) False.
(d) False.
(e) False.

A dentigerous cyst is invariably associated with an unerupted tooth. Unerupted teeth are associated with ameloblastomas. Dentigerous cysts are typically associated with the upper and lower third molars or the premolars in children. Impacted teeth are particularly associated with adenomatoid odontogenic tumours. Non-vital teeth are associated with radicular cysts, cementomas, and Garre's sclerosing osteomyelitis.

  (a) False.
       (b) True.
       (c) False.
       (d) True.
       (e) False.

Most ameloblastomas occur in the mandible, fewer in the maxilla. Nasolabial cysts occur in the soft tissues between the nose and upper lip and may cause adjacent maxillary bone resorption. Multiple dentigerous cysts occur in Gorlin's syndrome (also associated with multiple basal cell naevi, rib abnormalities and lamellar falx calcification). Carious teeth may be associated with periapical, periodontal or radicular cysts. Hyperparathyroidism and associated brown tumours may present as cystic lesions in the jaw.

  (a) True.
       (b) False.
       (c) True.
       (d) True.
       (e) True.

Recognised causes of generalised loss of the lamina dura are osteoporosis, hyperparathyroidism, Cushing's disease, osteomalacia, Paget's disease and scleroderma. Localised loss of the lamina dura may be caused by infection, tumours including multiple myeloma, metastases, Burkitt's lymphoma and Langerhans cell histiocytosis.

  (a) False.
       (b) False.
       (c) True.
       (d) False.
       (e) True.

The inferior alveolar nerve enters the mandible via the mandibular foramen and exits via the mental foramen. The muscles of mastication are generally innervated by the mandibular branch of the trigeminal nerve. CT scan is used to assess the height, width and contour of the alveolar process before dental implant placement. Mandibular fractures tend to be orientated parallel to the long axis of the roots of the teeth. Taste fibres from the anterior two-thirds of the tongue pass in the chorda tympani nerve, which is carried in the lingual nerve.

 A5   (a)   True.
(b)   False.
(c)   False.
(d)   False.
(e)   True.

Because of the variability in appearance of the mandible, diagnosis of mandibular osteomyelitis usually requires serial CT scanning to assess for progressive change. Bilateral mandibular fractures are commoner than unilateral because the mandible acts as a bony ring. The doses for an OPG and a bitewing radiograph are approximately 10–25 μSv and 5–10 μSv, respectively. If a bitewing film needs to be held still this should be done by the patient, not by the dentist or assistant.

Section 9

Head and neck

Q1 Are the following statements regarding thyroid carcinoma true or false?

(a) The most common subtype is follicular.
(b) Anaplastic carcinoma usually presents with local lymph node metastases.
(c) Medullary carcinoma is typically hyperdense on computed tomography (CT).
(d) Follicular carcinoma is often indistinguishable from benign follicular adenoma.
(e) Radiation-induced thyroid carcinoma peaks two to four years after exposure.

Q2 Are the following statements regarding thyroiditis true or false?

(a) In the early stages Hashimoto's thyroiditis is hyper-echogenic on ultrasound.
(b) In the late stages de Quervain's thyroiditis shows increased radioiodine uptake.
(c) Ultrasonography of acute suppurative thyroiditis may demonstrate an abscess.
(d) Hashimoto's thyroiditis is commoner in men than women.
(e) In late-stage Hashimoto's thyroiditis the thyroid may demonstrate acoustic shadowing.

Q3 Are the following statements regarding juvenile angiofibroma true or false?

(a) Although benign it often invades the sphenoid sinus.

151

(b)   Widening of the pterygopalatine fossa is a typical sign.
(c)   It is generally of high signal intensity on T1-weighted magnetic resonance imaging (MRI).
(d)   CT-guided biopsy is a good means of investigation.
(e)   Arterial supply is usually via the facial artery.

Q4   Are the following statements regarding fractures of the orbital floor true or false?

(a)   Orbital floor fractures are commoner than orbital roof fractures.
(b)   The medial rectus nerve may herniate through an orbital floor fracture.
(c)   Orbital floor and medial wall fractures rarely co-exist.
(d)   Orbital emphysema is almost always seen.
(e)   Absence of air-fluid level suggests that the fracture is old.

Q5   Are the following statements regarding epiglottitis true or false?

(a)   The peak age is 2 years.
(b)   The commonest causative organism is *Streptococcus*.
(c)   The hypopharynx typically appears narrowed.
(d)   Supine and erect plain films of the neck may be helpful.
(e)   Anteroposterior films are useful to diagnose croup.

Q6   Are the following statements regarding Graves' disease true or false?

(a)   The patient may not be hyperthyroid.
(b)   The most commonly affected muscle is the medial rectus.
(c)   Tendinous insertions are usually spared.
(d)   Intracranial herniation of fat is a strong predictor of ophthalmopathy.
(e)   Optic nerve crowding with effacement of perineural fat is a poor predictor of ophthalmopathy.

Q7   Are the following statements regarding glomus jugulare tumours true or false?

(a)   Glomus jugulare tumours usually arise in the pars nervosa of the jugular foramen.
(b)   Urinary catecholamine studies are required pre-embolisation.
(c)   The jugular vein is occasionally involved.
(d)   They classically present with deafness or tinnitus.
(e)   The differential for a vascular erosive mass includes haemangiopericytoma.

 Q8   Are the following statements regarding the salivary glands true or false?

(a)   Stones are commoner in the parotid gland than the submandibular gland.
(b)   Stensen's duct is narrower than Wharton's duct.
(c)   Sarcoid disease is associated with increased stone formation.
(d)   Painful enlargement of the parotid glands is seen in cirrhosis.
(e)   Chronic infection of the submandibular glands is recognised to mimic tumour.

 Q9   Are the following statements regarding Thornwaldt cysts true or false?

(a)   They occur in 1–5% of healthy adults.
(b)   They are low signal on T1-weighted MRI.
(c)   They may present with halitosis.
(d)   The differential diagnosis includes teratoma.
(e)   They are located between the superior and middle inferior constrictors in the midline.

Are the following statements regarding Le Fort fractures true or false?

(a) In a Le Fort I fracture the pterygoid plates are not fractured.
(b) Le Fort II fractures affect the medial and inferior orbits.
(c) The lateral orbit is not fractured in a Le Fort III.
(d) Le Fort I fractures affect the lower maxilla and not the orbits.
(e) Trimalar fractures affect the zygoma attachment to the frontal and sphenoid bones.

Answers

 (a) False.
(b) True.
(c) False.
(d) True.
(e) False.

The commonest subtype of thyroid carcinoma is papillary (60%), followed by follicular (20%), anaplastic (15%) and medullary (5%). Medullary carcinoma is typically hypodense since it does not concentrate iodine. Radiation-induced thyroid carcinoma peaks 10–20 years post exposure although cases have been reported 50 years post exposure.

 (a) False.
(b) True.
(c) True.
(d) True.
(e) True.

Hashimoto's thyroiditis is commoner in men than women. In the early stages the gland is hypoechoic and later it becomes fibrous, manifesting as hyperechoic and casting acoustic shadows. de Quervain's thyroiditis is more common in women, and usually follows an upper respiratory tract infection. On radioiodine nuclear medicine imaging, the thyroid is initially overactive (decreased uptake) and then underactive (increased uptake).

 (a) True.
(b) True.
(c) False.
(d) False.
(e) False.

Juvenile angiofibromas, although benign tend to invade local structures, especially the pterygopalatine fossa and sphenoid sinus. On MRI they are of intermediate signal intensity with areas of hypo-intensity. Arterial supply is via the maxillary artery, and because these tumours are highly vascular, biopsy is contraindicated.

 (a) True.
(b) True.
(c) False.
(d) False.
(e) True.

Although they are of the same thickness, the orbital floor fractures more frequently than the roof because of the infraorbital nerve and associated canal. The inferior rectus most commonly herniates through, then the inferior oblique and then the medial rectus. In 50% of cases, orbital floor and medial wall fractures co-exist. Orbital emphysema is thought to be rare because of the sealant effect of intraorbital fat.

 (a) False.
(b) True.
(c) False.
(d) False.
(e) True.

Epiglottitis is commoner after 3 years, peaking at 6 years of age in children. Young adults (aged 20–40 years) may also be affected. The commonest causative organism is *Haemophilus influenzae*. The hypopharynx typically appears ballooned. Supine films (including CT scanning) are contraindicated since they may precipitate acute respiratory obstruction. Croup occurs in a younger age group (less than 3 years) and anteroposterior films may demonstrate laryngeal 'steepling'.

 A6   (a) True.
        (b) False.
        (c) True.
        (d) True.
        (e) False.

The most commonly affected muscle in Graves' disease is the lateral rectus. Tendinous insertions are usually spared (in contrast to orbital pseudotumour). Intracranial herniation of fat (through the superior orbital fissure) and optic nerve crowding with effacement of perineural fat are strong predictors of ophthalmopathy, which may occur precipitately.

 A7   (a) False.
        (b) True.
        (c) False.
        (d) True.
        (e) True.

Glomus jugulare tumours usually arise in the pars vascularis. About 5% of tumours secrete catecholamines and so studies are required pre-embolisation. The jugular vein is almost always involved. The differential for a vascular erosive mass includes haemangiopericytoma, vascular metastasis, meningioma and angiofibroma.

 A8   (a) False.
        (b) True.
        (c) True.
        (d) False.
        (e) True.

Stones are thought to be commoner in the submandibular gland than the parotid gland because the saliva it produces is thicker, more alkaline and more mucinous. Sarcoid disease, hyperparathyroidism and Sjögren's syndrome are associated with increased stone formation. The enlargement of the parotid glands seen in cirrhosis (as well as diabetes, hypothyroidism and malnutrition) is usually painless. Chronic infection of the submandibular glands may cause firm focal masses referred to as Kuttner tumour.

A9　(a)　True.
　　(b)　False.
　　(c)　True.
　　(d)　True.
　　(e)　False.

Thornwaldt cysts occur in 1–5% of healthy adults and are remnants of a pharyngeal bursa which is retracted as the notochord ascends into the clivus. They are located in the midline above the superior constrictor muscles. They are typically high signal on T1- and T2-weighted MR images. They may present with halitosis, pain, discharge or nasal obstruction. The differential diagnosis includes teratoma and nasopharyngeal craniopharyngioma.

A10　(a)　False.
　　(b)　True.
　　(c)　False.
　　(d)　True.
　　(e)　True.

The pterygoid plates are not fractured in all Le Fort I fractures, which affect the lower maxilla and not the orbits. Le Fort II fractures affect the medial and inferior orbits. Le Fort III cross the lateral, inferior and medial walls of the orbit and cause craniofacial dislocation. Trimalar fractures affect the attachment of the zygoma to the maxilla, frontal and sphenoid bones.

Section 10

Genitourinary, adrenal and breast

Q1 Are the following statements regarding bladder cancer true or false?

(a) Invasion of the deep muscle wall constitutes T3a disease.
(b) Overstaging due to oedema post cystoscopy is a recognised pitfall.
(c) Tumour typically enhances on MR scanning.
(d) Calcification within the tumour is common.
(e) It is most common at the bladder trigone.

Q2 Are the following statements regarding testicular tumours true or false?

(a) The peak age for yolk sac tumours is 25–35 years.
(b) The commonest tumour type in undescended testes is teratoma.
(c) Epidermoid cysts are typically hyperechoic with acoustic shadowing.
(d) Tumours greater than 2 cm diameter are usually hypovascular.
(e) Patients with seminoma usually have normal serum alpha foetoprotein.

Q3 Are the following statements regarding testicular torsion true or false?

(a) It is commoner in patients with undescended testes.
(b) Operative correction within 24 hours gives a salvage rate of better than 75%.

159

(c)   Affected testes appear normal on grey scale ultrasound.
(d)   Nuclear medicine scan is highly sensitive.
(e)   Incomplete torsion may cause false negative Doppler flow studies.

(Q4)   Are the following statements regarding renal vein thrombosis true or false?

(a)   In longstanding cases the affected kidney is hypoechoic and enlarged.
(b)   The postpartum state is a recognised risk factor.
(c)   Intravenous urography (IVU) typically demonstrates a striated or dense nephrogram.
(d)   The proximal renal vein usually appears narrowed on ultrasonography.
(e)   Notching of the renal pelvis is seen in chronic cases.

(Q5)   Are the following statements regarding renal trauma true or false?

(a)   Enhancement of the renal periphery may be seen in shattered kidney.
(b)   The majority of renal injuries require surgical intervention.
(c)   If the kidneys fail to opacify on intravenous urography then catheter or CT angiography is indicated.
(d)   Apparent perirenal haematoma on CT may be due to pulsation artefact.
(e)   Renal contusion usually appears on CT as a high-density area.

(Q6)   Are the following statements regarding the anatomy of the kidney true or false?

(a)   The optimal plane for nephrostomy lies at the junction of the anterior third and posterior two-thirds of the kidney.
(b)   At the renal hilum, the artery lies anterior to the vein.

(c) In the neonate the kidneys are typically hypoechoic compared to liver and spleen.

(d) The column of Bertin represents the embryological fusion of anterior and posterior subkidneys.

(e) The column of Bertin is hypoechoic on ultrasound.

Q7   Are the following statements regarding intravenous urography (IVU) true or false?

(a) It is the radiologist's responsibility to assess renal function before performing IVU on patients currently taking Metformin.

(b) A normal serum creatinine level in the last 12 months is acceptable evidence of normal renal function.

(c) Any patient taking Metformin found to have abnormal renal function should have their drug history reviewed by the referring team.

(d) The presence of a known abdominal mass is a contraindication to compression in IVU.

(e) The right kidney may appear up to 2 cm larger than the left kidney.

Q8   Are the following statements regarding oncocytomas true or false?

(a) They usually present in patients less than 50 years old.

(b) Angiography typically demonstrates no arterio-venous shunting or contrast pooling.

(c) A central scar is seen in more than 50% of cases on CT.

(d) They frequently calcify.

(e) Percutaneous needle biopsy is unhelpful in diagnosis.

Q9   Are the following statements regarding angiomyolipomas true or false?

(a) They are seen in 20% of patients with tuberous sclerosis.

(b) They are commoner on the right side.

(c) They often present with haematuria.

(d) They are usually hypoechoic on ultrasound.
(e) Their risk of bleeding is approximately 90% at 4 cm.

Q10 Are the following statements regarding kidney and bladder MRI true or false?

(a) Columns of Bertin follow the signal intensity of renal cortex on all MR sequences.
(b) Renal cell carcinoma is often hypointense on T2-weighted images.
(c) In kidneys with fetal lobulation uniform cortical thickness is seen in post contrast images.
(d) In a normal distended bladder wall thickness may be up to 15 mm.
(e) In bladder cancer, enhancement after administration of intravenous contrast is delayed rather than immediate.

Q11 Are the following statements regarding urogenital malformations true or false?

(a) Pelvic kidneys are associated with an increased risk of hydronephrosis.
(b) In cross-fused ectopia the ectopic kidney usually lies inferiorly.
(c) Ureteric obstruction in horseshoe kidneys is commonly because of overlying veins.
(d) Congenital megaloureter is commoner in females.
(e) In bladder exstrophy the umbilicus is usually positioned high.

Q12 Are the following statements regarding MRI of the prostate gland true or false?

(a) Zonal anatomy is definable on T1-weighted images.
(b) The central zone is hypointense and the peripheral zone hyperintense on T2-weighted images.
(c) Müllerian duct cysts communicate with the posterior urethra.

(d) Benign prostatic hypertrophy may be heterogeneous or homogeneous in signal intensity.

(e) Prostate adenocarcinoma is frequently high signal on T2-weighted images.

(Q13) Are the following statements regarding prostate adeno-carcinoma true or false?

(a) Approximately 20% of patients with prostate cancer have a normal prostate specific antigen (PSA) level.

(b) For stage T2c tumour must be present in both lobes.

(c) Stage T3a tumour extends into seminal vesicles.

(d) Tumours are usually hyperechoic on transrectal ultra-sonography.

(e) MRI is highly sensitive for extracapsular extension.

(Q14) Are the following statements regarding urogenital anatomy true or false?

(a) The peripheral zone of the prostate is most extensive within the prostatic apex.

(b) The transitional zone of the prostate is most extensive within the midpart of the gland.

(c) The peripheral zone of the prostate increases in size with age.

(d) The central zone is located periurethrally.

(e) The dorsal component of the penis contains the paired corpora spongiosa.

(Q15) Are the following statements regarding the urethra true or false?

(a) The bulbous urethra traverses the urogenital diaphragm.

(b) The penile urethra contains the fossa navicularis.

(c) Urethrography should be avoided for a month follow-ing urethral instrumentation.

(d) Active urethritis is a contraindication to urethro-graphy.

(e) A 16F catheter is suitable for urethrography.

Q16 Are the following statements regarding testicular imaging true or false?

(a) Seminomas are low in signal intensity on T2-weighted MRI.
(b) 75% of testicular neoplasms are malignant.
(c) A significant proportion of metastases to the testes arise from the prostate gland.
(d) An epidermoid cyst with whorled or onion skin appearance does not require surgery as long as imaging follow up demonstrates no change.
(e) Any mass or vascularity associated with an intensely echogenic epidermoid cyst is an indication for surgery.

 Q17 Are the following statements regarding anatomy of the testes true or false?

(a) The spermatic cord carries the pampiniform plexus.
(b) Testicular cysts are seen in up to 1% of normal testes.
(c) The appendix testis is found at the lower pole of the testis.
(d) A small hydrocele can be seen in 10–15% of normal patients.
(e) The tunica albuginea invaginates into the testis at the mediastinum testis.

 Q18 Are the following statements regarding the adrenal glands true or false?

(a) On ultrasound the left adrenal is more frequently visualised than the right.
(b) On ultrasound the normal adrenal gland thickness is up to 2 cm.
(c) The outer adrenal cortex is responsible for sex hormone production.
(d) On CT visualisation of the left adrenal is approximately 100%.
(e) The normal adrenal gland may be up to 5 cm long.

Are the following statements regarding adrenal masses true or false?

(a) A mass up to 3 cm in size is malignant in approximately 10–15% of cases.
(b) An attenuation value of less than 10 Hounsfield Units on unenhanced CT means that the lesion must be an adenoma.
(c) An attenuation value of less than 25 Hounsfield Units 15 minutes after enhancement on CT means that the lesion is almost certainly benign.
(d) Adrenal adenomas may calcify.
(e) Phaeochromocytoma is a recognised cause of bilateral large adrenals.

 Are the following statements regarding MRI of the adrenal glands true or false?

(a) In phase images show signal dropout in benign adenomas.
(b) Benign adenomas enhance more homogeneously than metastases.
(c) Metastases are usually darker on T2-weighted images than adenomas.
(d) Small adrenal masses are optimally demonstrated with T1-weighted fat saturated sequences.
(e) Sagittal images are generally found more helpful in defining adrenal masses than coronal.

 Are the following statements regarding mammography true or false?

(a) The typical dose of a mammogram is 0.2 mGy.
(b) A double-coated film is used to improve detection of microcalcifications.
(c) A focal spot of 0.01 mm is usually used.
(d) Compression helps reduce image blurring.
(e) A grid increases the dose.

Q22 Are the following statements regarding breast anatomy true or false?

(a) Each breast is composed of 15–20 lobes.
(b) Each main lactiferous duct is 2–5 mm in diameter.
(c) The normal skin thickness is up to 5 mm.
(d) Lymph may drain directly to subscapular nodes.
(e) Axillary nodes drain 50% of lymph from the breast.

Q23 Are the following statements regarding breast micro-calcifications true or false?

(a) Malignant microcalcifications are usually about 1 mm in diameter.
(b) Linear/branching pattern is a benign feature.
(c) Solid rod-shaped calcifications are a benign feature.
(d) Malignant microcalcifications can remain stable for 5 years.
(e) Concentration of more than five microcalcifications per square cm is a benign feature.

Q24 Are the following statements regarding ultrasound of breast nodules true or false?

(a) A single malignant feature may be seen in an ultra-sonically benign nodule.
(b) A lesion being taller than it is wide is a benign feature.
(c) Acoustic shadowing behind a lesion is a malignant feature.
(d) Presence of multiple small lobulations (microlobulation) is a malignant feature.
(e) Marked hypoechogenicity is a benign feature.

Q25 Are the following statements regarding mammography of breast nodules true or false?

(a) Well-defined nodules less than 1 cm in diameter are unlikely to be malignant.
(b) A lobulated outline is more suspicious than oval.

(c) Intramammary lymph nodes usually occur in the lower outer quadrant.
(d) Fat containing lesions are sometimes malignant.
(e) Sebaceous cysts are usually high density.

Q26 Are the following statements regarding breast carcinoma true or false?

(a) Medullary carcinoma is the fastest growing type.
(b) Mucinous/colloid carcinoma is usually well circumscribed.
(c) Papillary carcinoma does not demonstrate acoustic enhancement.
(d) Low-grade tubal carcinoma is bilateral in one-third of patients.
(e) Medullary carcinoma usually shows some through transmission ultrasonically.

Q27 Are the following statements regarding MRI of the breast true or false?

(a) Silicone is high signal on T2 imaging.
(b) The standard protocol does not require intravenous contrast.
(c) Carcinomas tend to enhance more than benign lesions with contrast.
(d) MRI is more sensitive than ultrasound for detecting implant rupture.
(e) MRI is of less value in patients with multicentric breast cancer.

Q28 Are the following statements regarding benign dense asymmetric breast tissue true or false?

(a) Typically evolves over time.
(b) May contain fat.
(c) Is commonest in the lower outer quadrant.
(d) May be palpable.
(e) Is seen in 3% of breasts.

Are the following statements regarding breast lesions true or false?

(a) Surgical scar tissue may appear spiculated for up to 3 years.
(b) Post radiation scar may appear spiculated.
(c) Diffuse skin thickening is a recognised sign of breast cancer.
(d) Skin retraction is due to shortening of Cooper's ligaments.
(e) Rim calcification is atypical of fat necrosis.

 Are the following statements regarding Paget's disease of the nipple true or false?

(a) Usually presents with a palpable mass.
(b) May present with nipple eczema.
(c) Is typically associated with large calcifications.
(d) Ductography often reveals a dilated duct.
(e) Mammography is positive in 50% of cases.

Answers

  (a) True.
(b) True.
(c) False.
(d) False.
(e) False.

In bladder cancer stage T1 disease involves mucosa and submucosal; T2 disease invades the superficial muscle layer; T3a disease extends into deep muscle layer; T3b involves perivesical organs such as the bladder and rectum; and T4b disease constitutes invasion of the abdominal or pelvic wall. Typically tumour fails to enhance with contrast. Calcification is rare ($\sim$1%). Bladder malignancy is commonest at the sidewalls and in bladder diverticula.

A2   (a)   False.
         (b)   False.
         (c)   True.
         (d)   False.
         (e)   True.

The peak age for yolk sac tumours is before puberty. Seminoma is the commonest tumour type in undescended testes and unlike teratoma is associated with a normal serum alpha foetoprotein. Small tumours (<1.5 cm) are usually hypovascular; large tumours (>2 cm) are usually hypervascular.

 A3   (a)   True.
         (b)   False.
         (c)   True.
         (d)   True.
         (e)   True.

Testicular torsion is 10 times commoner in patients with un-descended testes. Testicular salvage rates decrease after 6 hours to 75% and after 12 hours to 20%. Doppler flow studies of the spermatic cord and nuclear medicine imaging with pertechnetate scan are highly sensitive. Spontaneous detorsion and incomplete torsion are recognised causes of false negative Doppler flow studies.

 A4   (a)   False.
         (b)   True.
         (c)   True.
         (d)   False.
         (e)   True.

In acute cases the affected kidney is hypoechoic and enlarged; in chronic cases the affected kidney is hyperechoic and small. Hyper-coagulable states are a risk factor and include dehydration, malignancy and nephrotic syndrome. IVU demonstrates poor opacification with a prolonged or striated nephrogram. The proximal renal vein usually appears dilated on ultrasonography. Ureteric or renal pelvis notching is seen in chronic cases due to formation of collaterals (which may also be visualised on cross-sectional imaging).

(a) True.
(b) False.
(c) True.
(d) False.
(e) False.

Enhancement of the renal periphery may be seen in shattered kidney due to perfusion by collateral vessels. Most renal injuries can be simply imaged and observed. Apparent perirenal haematoma on CT may be due to respiratory artefact. Renal contusion usually appears on CT as a low-density area.

(a) False.
(b) False.
(c) False.
(d) False.
(e) False.

The renal artery divides into major ventral and dorsal branches, which creates a zone of relative avascularity (known as Brödel's line) lying just posterior to the lateral convex border of the kidney, at the junction of the anterior two-thirds and posterior one-third of the kidney. Traversing this avascular region minimises bleeding complications from nephrostomy. The ventral renal artery branches lie between the renal vein and ureter, the vein being in front, the ureter behind; the dorsal branch usually lies behind the ureter. In the neonate the kidneys are typically hyperechoic compared to liver and spleen (since they have a relatively higher proportion of glomeruli in the renal cortex). The column of Bertin represents the embryological fusion of superior and inferior subkidneys, and runs obliquely and forwards, appearing as a hyperechoic line.

(a) False.
(b) True.
(c) True.
(d) True.
(e) False.

Current guidelines with regard to Metformin-induced lactic acidosis and contrast medium agents are available on the Royal College of

Radiologists website, www.rcr.ac.uk. The referring clinician should take responsibility for assessing the patients' renal function, either by checking the serum creatinine or accepting a normal level within the past year. The Radiology Department should inform the referring clinician of the timing of the investigation to enable this to occur. As the British Diabetic Association states that Metformin is contraindicated in the presence of abnormal renal function, it is suggested that such patients who require intravascular contrast examinations should have their drug history reviewed by the appropriate physician to ensure suitability of the drug regimen. Contraindications to abdominal compression include evidence of obstruction on the 5-minute image, abdominal aortic aneurysm or some other abdominal mass, recent abdominal surgery or severe abdominal pain, suspected urinary tract trauma, and presence of urinary diversion or a renal transplant. On IVU the left kidney may appear up to 2 cm larger than the right kidney (due to radiographic magnification).

 (a) False.
(b) True.
(c) False.
(d) False.
(e) True.

The median age for presentation of oncocytomas is 65, although the age range is wide. The presence of arterio-venous shunting, contrast pooling or renal vein invasion is more suggestive of renal cell carcinoma than oncocytoma. The central scar is seen in 20–40% of cases. Calcification is rare. Percutaneous needle biopsy is unreliable in establishing a diagnosis; removal and examination of the whole kidney is recommended since renal cell carcinomas may have areas of oncocytic transformation.

 (a) False.
(b) True.
(c) True.
(d) False.
(e) False.

Angiomyolipomas are seen in 70–80% of patients with tuberous sclerosis and are usually large, bilateral and multiple in contrast to sporadic cases. They may bleed profusely, and can present with retroperitoneal haemorrhage or haematuria (in 40% of cases). They are typically hyperechoic on ultrasound due to their fat content. Their risk of bleeding increases with size and is 50% at 4 cm.

(A10) (a) True.
      (b) False.
      (c) True.
      (d) False.
      (e) True.

Columns of Bertin follow the signal intensity of renal cortex on all MR sequences, both pre and post contrast. Renal cell carcinoma is usually hyperintense on T2-weighted images, although it may rarely be isointense. Uniform cortical thickness is seen in post contrast images in kidneys with fetal lobulations, which helps exclude a renal mass. On MRI 2–8 mm is usually taken as the limits of wall thickness in a distended bladder.

(A11) (a) True.
      (b) True.
      (c) False.
      (d) True.
      (e) False.

Pelvic kidneys are associated with an increased risk of hydro-nephrosis because of an abnormal insertion of the ureter into the renal pelvis. Ureteric obstruction in horseshoe kidneys is commonly because of overlying arteries. Congenital megaloureter is commoner in females and on the left side and is due to an aperistaltic segment of ureter usually in the juxtavesical region. In bladder exstrophy the umbilicus is usually positioned low, and there is often diastasis of the pubic symphysis.

(A12) (a) False.
      (b) True.
      (c) False.

(d) True.
(e) False.

Zonal anatomy is indistinguishable on T1-weighted images. Müllerian duct cysts do not communicate with the posterior urethra (unlike utricular cysts), although they do connect with the verumontanum via a stalk. Benign prostatic hypertrophy is moderate to high signal on T2-weighted images and may be heterogeneous or homogeneous. Prostate adenocarcinoma is usually low signal on T2-weighted images and occasionally intermediate signal, with high signal tumours only seen rarely; these are usually found to have prominent mucinous components on histopathological examination.

 (a) True.
(b) True.
(c) False.
(d) False.
(e) True.

Approximately 20% of prostate cancers do not secrete prostate specific antigen (PSA). Stage T2a tumour involves up to half of one lobe, T2b involves more than half of one lobe, and T2c represents tumour in both lobes. Stage T3a tumour indicates unilateral extracapsular extension, T3b bilateral extension, and stage T3c represents invasion into seminal vesicles. Almost two-thirds of tumours are hypoechoic on transrectal ultrasonography, one-third isoechoic and a small proportion (~2%) hyperechoic. MRI has a sensitivity of 90% for extracapsular extension.

 (a) True.
(b) False.
(c) False.
(d) True.
(e) False.

The transitional zone of the prostate is most extensive within the base of the gland and increases in size with age. The dorsal component of the penis contains the paired corpora cavernosa.

(a) False.
  (b) True.
  (c) False.
  (d) True.
  (e) False.

The membranous urethra traverses the urogenital diaphragm. Urethrography should be avoided during active, untreated urethritis, and should be postponed for one week following urethral instrumentation. Water-soluble contrast media is injected through a small (size 8) Foley catheter inserted under sterile conditions.

 (a) True.
  (b) False.
  (c) True.
  (d) False.
  (e) True.

Seminomas are low in signal intensity on T2-weighted MRI and enhance less than normal surrounding testis. 95% of testicular neoplasms are malignant. Metastases to the testes are commoner than germ cell tumours in patients over 50 years of age. Primary sites include prostate, lung, kidney and gastrointestinal tract (in descending order of frequency). Current recommendations are that most types of epidermoid cyst are enucleated; only those which are intensively echogenic with no associated mass or vascularity may be followed up.

 (a) True.
  (b) False.
  (c) False.
  (d) True.
  (e) True.

The spermatic cord carries the testicular and cremasteric arteries, the pampiniform plexus, nerves and lymph vessels as well as the vas deferens. Testicular cysts are seen in up to 10% of normal testes. The appendix testis is a remnant of the paramesonephric duct at the upper pole of the testis.

(a) False.
  (b) False.
  (c) False.
  (d) True.
  (e) True.

On ultrasound the right adrenal is more frequently visualised than the left (quoted visibility: right adrenal 80%, left adrenal 45%). The normal adrenal gland thickness is up to 1 cm on ultrasound. The normal adrenal gland may be up to 5 × 3 × 1 cm.

  (a) True.
  (b) False.
  (c) True.
  (d) True.
  (e) False.

An attenuation value of less than 10 Hounsfield Units on un-enhanced CT means that the lesion is almost certainly benign (96%). Other recognised causes of bilateral large adrenals include: hyperplasia, haemorrhage, Hodgkin's disease, tuberculosis, histo-plasmosis and metastases.

  (a) False.
  (b) True.
  (c) False.
  (d) True.
  (e) True.

Out of phase images show signal dropout in benign adenomas because of intracytoplasmic lipid. Benign adenomas enhance more homogeneously and for less time than metastases. Metastases are usually brighter on T2-weighted images than adenomas. Sagittal coronal images are generally found more helpful in defining adrenal masses than coronal because there is less partial volume effect from adjacent structures.

A21 (a) False.
  (b) False.
  (c) False.

(d) True.
(e) True.

The typical dose of a mammogram is approximately 2 mGy, which carries a risk of inducing fatal cancer of about 20/million at age 30–50 years. A single-coated film is used to prevent parallax. A focal spot of 0.3 mm or less is used, with a focal spot of 0.1 mm for spot views. Breast compression helps reduce image blurring by causing immobilisation, reducing object-film distance, and helps equalise tissue thickness. A grid or air gap is routinely used to improve contrast but increases dose.

  (a) True.
(b) True.
(c) False.
(d) True.
(e) False.

Each breast is composed of 15–20 lobes, each connecting to a main lactiferous duct which is 2–5 mm in diameter. Normal skin thickness is 1–3 mm. More than 75% of lymph drainage is to the axillary nodes with most of the rest to the parasternal nodes, although some also passes to other local nodes including the subscapular.

  (a) False.
(b) False.
(c) True.
(d) True.
(e) False.

Malignant microcalcifications are usually less than 0.5 mm in diameter and can remain stable for 5 years or more. Benign morphologies include: smooth round, solid/lucent-centred spheres, crescents, parallel tracks, solid rod-shaped, and eggshell. Malignant morphologies include: vermicular shape, linear/branching and variation in size of microcalcifications. Concentration of less than four per square cm is a benign feature.

  (a) False.
(b) False.

    (c)   True.
    (d)   True.
    (e)   False.

Any single malignant feature renders any nodule ultrasonically malignant. Malignant features on ultrasound include being taller than wide, spiculation, angular margins, extreme hypoechogenicity, posterior acoustic shadowing, punctuate calcifications, micro-lobulation, and radial extension.

 (A25)   (a)   True.
         (b)   True.
         (c)   False.
         (d)   False.
         (e)   True.

In descending order of malignant potential, outlines are ranked irregular, lobulated, oval and round. Intramammary lymph nodes usually occur in the upper outer quadrant. Fat containing lesions are never malignant. Sebaceous cysts, simple cysts and abscesses are often high density with a halo sign.

 (A26)   (a)   True.
         (b)   True.
         (c)   False.
         (d)   True.
         (e)   True.

Medullary, mucinous/colloid, and papillary subtypes each account for ~2% of breast cancer; tubal carcinoma accounts for 6–8%. Medullary carcinoma is the fastest growing type; it is soft, demon-strating through transmission ultrasonically and may be mistaken for fibroadenoma. Mucinous/colloid carcinoma is usually well circumscribed and may demonstrate punctuate calcifications. Pap-illary carcinoma demonstrates acoustic enhancement. Low-grade tubal carcinoma is bilateral in one-third of patients; high grade is bilateral in 1 in 300 patients.

 (A27)   (a)   True.
         (b)   False.

   (c) True.
   (d) True.
   (e) False.

Silicone is low signal on T1 and high signal on T2. Most standard protocols require fat suppressed dynamic contrast enhanced imaging; most carcinomas enhance within the first 3 minutes. MRI is more sensitive than ultrasound for detecting implant rupture (90–95% versus 70–75%), and is particularly useful in patients with dense breasts and multicentric breast cancer which may appear super-imposed on mammography.

A28   (a) False.
      (b) True.
      (c) False.
      (d) False.
      (e) True.

Benign dense asymmetric breast tissue is commonest in the upper outer quadrant and may contain fat, but should not be associated with palpable mass, calcification or architectural distortion. It should not evolve over time and is seen in 3% of breasts.

A29   (a) False.
      (b) True.
      (c) True.
      (d) True.
      (e) False.

Surgical scar tissue may appear spiculated for up to 1 year, and post radiation scar for up to 3 years. Rim calcification is typical of fat necrosis. Diffuse skin thickening is a sign of inflammatory breast cancer.

A30   (a) False.
      (b) True.
      (c) False.
      (d) True.
      (e) True.

Paget's disease usually presents with nipple discharge or eczema, and occasionally with a retroareolar soft tissue mass. Mammography is positive in 50% of cases and reveals microcalcifications in a linear distribution. Ductography often reveals a dilated duct.

Bibliography

General preclinical text

- Francis IS, Aviv RI, Dick EA *et al.* (eds) (1999) *Fundamental Aspects of Radiology*. Remedica, London.

Anatomy

- Ryan S, McNicholas M and Eustace S (2004) *Anatomy for Diagnostic Imaging* (2e). WB Saunders, Edinburgh.

Physics

- Farr RF and Allisy-Roberts PJ (1997) *Physics for Medical Imaging*. WB Saunders, London.

Techniques

- Chapman S and Nakileny R (2001) *A Guide to Radiological Procedures* (4e). WB Saunders, Edinburgh.
- Whitehouse GH and Worthington BS (1996) *Techniques in Diagnostic Imaging*. Blackwell Science, Oxford.

General clinical texts and atlases

- Dahnert W (2003) *Radiology Review Manual* (5e). Lippincott, Williams & Wilkins, Philadelphia.

- Chapman S and Nakielny R (2001) *Aids to Radiological Differential Diagnoses* (4e). WB Saunders, Edinburgh.
- Grainger RG, Allison DJ, Adam A *et al.* (2001) *Diagnostic Radiology: a textbook of medical imaging* (4e). Churchill Livingstone, London.
- Eisenberg R (2003) *Clinical Imaging: an atlas of differential diagnosis* (4e). Lippincott, Williams & Wilkins, Philadelphia.
- Meire HB, Cosgrove D, Dewbury K *et al.* (2001) *Abdominal and General Ultrasound* (2e). Churchill Livingstone, London.
- Wegener OH (1993) *Whole Body Computed Tomography* (2e). Blackwell Scientific, Boston.

Specialised texts

- Carty H (ed) (1999) *Emergency Pediatric Radiology*. Springer, Berlin.
- Osborn AG (1994) *Diagnostic Neuroradiology*. Mosby, St Louis.
- Rogers LF (ed) (2002) *Radiology of Skeletal Trauma* (3e). Churchill Livingstone, New York.
- Resnick D and Kang HS (1997) *Internal Derangements of Joints*. WB Saunders, Philadelphia.
- Ansell G, Betmann MA, Kaufmann JA *et al.* (eds) (1996) *Complications in Diagnostic Imaging and Interventional Radiology* (3e). Blackwell Science, Cambridge, MA.
- Hricak H and Carrington BM (1991) *MRI of the Pelvis*. Martin Dunitz, London.
- Brady TJ, Grist TM, Westra S *et al.* (2002) *Pocket Radiologist. Cardiac: top 100 diagnoses*. WB Saunders, Philadelphia.
- Thrall JH and Ziessman HA (2001) *Nuclear Medicine: the requisites* (2e). Mosby, St Louis.
- Armstrong P, Wilson A, Dee P *et al.* (2000) *Imaging of Diseases of the Chest* (3e). Mosby, London.
- Husband J and Reznek R (eds) (2004) *Imaging in Oncology* (2e). Taylor and Francis, London.
- Kessel D and Robertson I (2002) *Interventional Radiology: a survival guide*. Churchill Livingstone, Edinburgh.

Journals

- Recent editions of *Clinical Radiology*, *Radiology* and *Radiographics*, especially review articles.

Index

(q) refer to question locators; (a) refer to answer locators.

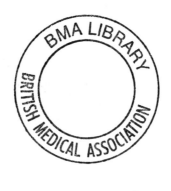